James Lloyd is a barrister at Mountford Chambers and Deputy Head of its Regulatory Practice Group. He practises in professional discipline and regulatory law. He regularly acts in fitness to practise proceedings, related appeals and judicial reviews for both registrants and regulators.

A Practical Guide to Proceedings Before the Nursing and Midwifery Council (NMC)

A Practical Guide to Proceedings Before the Nursing and Midwifery Council (NMC)

James Lloyd
Barrister, Lincoln's Inn
LL.B (Hons) (Newc)

Law Brief Publishing

Published 2026 by Law Brief Publishing, an imprint of Law Brief Publishing Ltd
30 The Parks
Minehead
Somerset
TA24 8BT

www.lawbriefpublishing.com

Paperback: 978-1-918241-22-8

PREFACE

I have written this book because Nursing and Midwifery Council proceedings are too often experienced as disorientating, intimidating and unsettling by those who encounter them.

In my own practice, I have seen too many registrants and witnesses emerge from the process shocked, not simply by the outcome but by the experience itself. Sadly, that shock is often accompanied by a loss of confidence in the regulator. In many cases, it does not arise because the process is inherently unfair, but because those involved do not understand, at a conceptual level, what the regulator is there to do. Expectations formed by employment processes, criminal proceedings or civil litigation are carried into a regulatory setting that operates on different principles, for different purposes.

For registrants, the fitness to practise process can feel opaque and overwhelming. For witnesses and employers, it can appear disconnected from familiar workplace procedures. For lawyers who do not practise regularly in FTP proceedings, it can seem procedurally unfamiliar and, at times, counter-intuitive. Yet beneath that surface complexity sits a surprisingly coherent statutory framework.

The Nursing and Midwifery Council is not an employment tribunal, nor is it a civil or criminal court. Its role is regulatory and protective. Fitness to practise proceedings are not brought to punish, even though their consequences are often serious and life-changing. They exist to protect the public, to maintain confidence in the professions, and to uphold proper professional standards. When those objectives are clearly understood, the structure of the process, and many of the decisions taken within it, make much more sense.

This book is written principally with practitioners in mind. Too often, lawyers approach NMC proceedings through the lens of criminal or civil litigation, importing an adversarial approach replete with assumptions about proof, procedure, evidence and outcome that do not sit comfortably within a regulatory scheme. While there are many points of overlap, professional discipline is a distinct area of law with its own statutory foundations, judgement patterns and public interest focus. Failing to recognise those nuances can manifest in misjudged strategy and unnecessary frustration for clients.

I cannot offer tactical shortcuts or a checklist for success. What this publication seeks to do instead is to provide a clear introduction to the statutory scheme governing NMC proceedings, to explain how the process operates in practice, and to help practitioners, registrants and others approach these proceedings with a clearer understanding of the regulatory purpose and the legal framework within which decisions are made.

At its best, professional regulation promotes safe practice and public confidence while treating individuals fairly. Achieving that balance is not always straightforward. My hope is that this book helps those working within the NMC's regulatory framework to approach proceedings with greater clarity, confidence and understanding, and to see not only how the process operates, but why it is designed in the way it is.

I am indebted to my colleagues at Mountford Chambers, whose collective expertise has shaped my practice over many years, and to the many practitioners and panel members I have encountered across fitness to practise proceedings, from whom I have learnt as much in disagreement and in accord. I am particularly grateful to the countless legal assessors who, with patience and precision, have corrected my occasional folly. I also thank Tim and Garry at Law Brief Publishing for their faith and patience throughout the development of this, my first published work.

Finally, I am asked to declare that to the best of my knowledge, matters of law stated in this publication are correct and up to date as of 18 January 2026.

James M. Lloyd
London
February 2026

CONTENTS

CHAPTER ONE

AN INTRODUCTION TO THE NURSING AND MIDWIFERY COUNCIL

1 **The Nursing and Midwifery Council**

1.1 The Nursing and Midwifery Council (NMC) is the statutory regulator for nurses, midwives and nursing associates in the United Kingdom. It is a creature of statute, entrusted by Parliament with responsibility for regulating professions whose work engages directly with patient safety, vulnerability and public confidence in healthcare services. The NMC's overarching objective is the protection of the public. That is not a corporate slogan; it is the guiding principle which governs how the NMC exercises its functions, how panels approach the determination of allegations, and how decisions are scrutinised by the courts.

1.2 The NMC is not a professional body, a representative organisation or an advocate for registrants in any traditional sense. Nor is it an employment tribunal or a forum for resolving workplace disputes. Its function is to oversee the profession as a whole, to secure public safety and confidence. The distinction matters. Many of the tensions that arise when registrants encounter the NMC's fitness to practise process stem from an understandable, but legally incorrect, assumption that the regulator is an extension of their employer, or a body designed to vindicate or punish. It is neither. It is a statutory creature responsible for controlling access to, and continued participation in, a regulated profession, in the public interest.

1.3 The NMC regulates the right to practise, not the right to be employed. The two often overlap in practice, particularly in the NHS, and a single set of facts can generate both employer action and regulatory action. They are nonetheless distinct jurisdictions, with different purposes, different tests and different outcomes.

1.4 For a reader approaching NMC proceedings for the first time, it is therefore useful to keep three propositions at the forefront of mind from the outset.

1.4.1 First, the framework is statutory. The NMC can act only where the statutory scheme permits it to act, and it must act in accordance with that scheme. The boundaries of the NMC's powers have been set by Parliament, though operationally panels enjoy broad case management discretion: familiarity with the statutory scheme, fitness to practise rules and standards is essential.

1.4.2 Second, the framework is protective. Fitness to practise proceedings are not brought to punish, even though they often have severe and punitive consequences. They are brought to protect the public, to maintain confidence in the professions, and to uphold proper standards. These aims percolate through all decision making, particularly during the fitness to practise process.

1.4.3 Third, the framework is public law in character. The NMC, and the panels which exercise its adjudicatory functions, are subject to the supervisory jurisdiction of the High Court. Decisions must be lawful, fair, reasoned and proportionate.

2 Statutory footing and regulatory purpose

2.1 The NMC's authority is conferred by the Nursing and Midwifery Order 2001 (the 2001 Order).[1] The 2001 Order establishes the NMC, creates and governs the register, and sets out the machinery through which regulation operates. It provides the framework for standard-setting, education and registration decisions, and fitness to practise. In that sense, it provides both the foundation and the boundary of the NMC's jurisdiction. The 2001 Order also defines the regulator's purpose. Articles 3(4) and 3(4A) state that the overarching objective of the NMC is the protection of the public, pursued through protecting, promoting and maintaining the health, safety and wellbeing of the public; promoting and maintaining public confidence in the professions regulated under the Order; and promoting and maintaining proper professional standards and conduct for registrants.

2.2 The statutory footing has two immediate consequences.

2.2.1 The NMC may act only within the powers conferred by Parliament. The NMC does not have a free-standing discretion to intervene whenever concerns are raised, however serious, emotive or politically charged. The statutory scheme defines the circumstances in which concerns may be investigated and, if appropriate, prosecuted. Where those gateways are not engaged, the NMC has no jurisdiction to proceed.

2.2.2 The NMC must exercise its powers for the purposes for which Parliament granted them. Regulatory power is not available as a means to resolve workplace

[1] SI 2002/253

disputes, to award compensation, to attribute blame for systemic service failure, or to "send a message" untethered to the statutory objectives. Where those objectives require intervention, the NMC is expected to act; where they do not, the statutory scheme provides no authority for intervention.

2.3 The NMC's functions are not limited to fitness to practise. Its remit is concerned with entry into a regulated profession, continued inclusion on the register, and the maintenance of professional standards across a working life. The NMC's regulatory duties therefore fall under three broad areas.

2.4 Standard-setting is one area. The NMC sets professional standards of conduct and performance for registrants, and educational standards for those seeking entry to the register. Those standards provide the normative yardstick against which allegations are assessed and suitability to practise assessed. They also influence the professional culture in which healthcare is delivered, by establishing what the regulator expects as a minimum. The NMC produces a wealth of guidance to registrants on professional conduct and the application of those standards. Registrants are expected to act in accordance with both the standards and the guidance, with the latter formally being instructive.

2.5 Registration control is the next. The register is not merely a list, but the legal instrument through which the state (by delegation) controls who may practise as a nurse, midwife or nursing associate. Entry decisions, restoration decisions and the maintenance of registration through revalidation are state-mandated controls of the utmost importance. Integrity of the register is a matter of public protection, and actions which undermine that integrity (for example, non-disclosure of criminal convictions or practising when registration has lapsed) are treated as among the most serious categories of misconduct.

2.6 Linked to, but distinct from those areas, is the the fitness to practise (FTP) process. This is the enforcement jurisdiction through which the regulator determines whether a registrant should remain on the register and, if so, whether their registration should be restricted. The FTP process is a further mechanism by which the regulator can declare and uphold proper professional standards.

3 Scope of regulation

3.1 The NMC regulates three professions: nurses, midwives and nursing associates. Only individuals whose names appear on the NMC register may practise in the protected roles conferred by registration. Regulation is therefore anchored in status: the holding of registration. That is why the NMC's jurisdiction follows the registrant across settings and roles.

3.2 The scope of regulation is wide. It applies across all fields of nursing and midwifery and across all sectors in which nurses, midwives and nursing associates practise or hold themselves out as entitled to practise: the NHS, private healthcare, social care, education, agency work, consultancy, and independent practice. It applies irrespective of seniority or job title. A registrant in a senior management role is not insulated from regulation on the basis that they no longer provide direct clinical care. Professional trustworthiness is not a clinical-only concept. Integrity, safeguarding judgement, and the ability to act professionally are relevant across roles. The scope of regulation also stretches into the private lives of registrants where conduct outside the workplace has the propensity to bring the profession into disrepute.

3.3 The NMC regulates individuals, not institutions. Employers, trusts, care homes, commissioning bodies and NHS England are not regulated by the NMC as such. The NMC's concern is the professional status of the individual registrant. That distinction is not pedantry. It explains why the NMC cannot determine employment disputes, award compensation, nor direct employers as to disciplinary outcomes. It also goes some way to explain conceptually why employer findings are not admissible in fitness to practise proceedings; they are not determinative of regulatory outcomes.

3.4 Protected titles are a familiar feature of statutory schemes and the NMC is no different. The titles "Registered Nurse", "Midwife", "Nursing Associate" and "Specialist Community Public Health Nurse" are protected in law and may only be used by those properly registered, with related criminal offences attaching to the misuse of these specific titles and functions. By contrast, "nurse" is not, in itself, a protected title, which means that in ordinary language the term is widely used while, as a matter of law, one could currently describe oneself and indeed practise as a "nurse" without registration, subject to the offence provisions in Article 44. This position has attracted criticism and ongoing policy attention, including the government's announcement in July 2025 of an intention to strengthen nursing title protection by closing this loophole. Whether those proposals translate into legislation remains a matter of statutory change rather than regulatory discretion.

3.5 Internationally qualified applicants sit within the same public protection scheme. The register is a UK register, and admission to it requires the NMC to be satisfied that an applicant meets the relevant UK standards. The detail of how the NMC assesses international qualifications and competence is largely set out in the NMC's published standards and registration guidance rather than in the 2001 Order itself, but the legal point remains: without registration there is no entitlement to practise in the protected roles.

3.6 Temporary or emergency registration powers are also part of the landscape and were used to great effect during the coronavirus period. Legislative mechanisms for temporary registration in emergencies involving loss of human life or human illness are reflected in consolidated legislative texts and the broader scheme of amendments: the register is a statutory tool capable of being adapted in exceptional circumstances to address public need while retaining a regulatory framework for standards and accountability.

4 The Register

4.1 The NMC maintains a single professional register, but that register is divided into distinct fields of practice. The structure reflects the reality that nursing and midwifery comprise distinct professional disciplines, each with their own education routes, standards of proficiency, and scopes of practice.

4.2 The legislative framework governing the register is set out in the 2001 Order (principally, Articles 5 and 6) together with its associated statutory instruments, and applies UK-wide. The 2001 Order requires the regulator to establish and maintain a register and to determine the standards of proficiency necessary for admission to the different parts of that register. It further provides that the register be divided into separate parts, each bearing a title which reflects the qualifications, education, or training required to entry the respective part. Registration on a particular part of the register entitles a practitioner to use the corresponding protected professional title.

4.3 Article 44 of the 2001 Order makes it a criminal offence for a person (with an intent to deceive) to: falsely represent themselves as being registered; claim registration in a part of the register to which they are not entitled; use a protected title unlawfully; or misrepresent their nursing or midwifery qualifications.

4.4 The division of the register flowing from the 2001 Order underpins all regulatory decision-making. In fitness to practise proceedings, panels must assess conduct, competence, and impairment by reference to the registrant's registered field or fields. It is not appropriate to judge a mental health nurse by adult nursing standards, or vice versa, unless the registrant is dual-registered and the factual matrix properly engages both parts of the register.

4.5 The register is divided into the following fields and parts:

Adult nursing

4.5.1 Adult nursing is the field concerned with the care of adults with physical health needs. It encompasses acute, chronic, and long-term conditions and is practised across hospital, community, and specialist services.

4.5.2 Registrants in this field are trained primarily in physical assessment, clinical reasoning, medicines management, and the delivery of evidence-based care for physical illness and injury. Their competence is assessed by reference to adult nursing standards and proficiencies, not by reference to other nursing disciplines.

4.5.3 On the register, these practitioners are recorded as Registered Nurse (Adult).

Mental health nursing

4.5.4 Mental health nursing is a distinct field focused on the care of people experiencing mental illness, psychological distress, and associated behavioural or emotional difficulties. Practice is centred on therapeutic engagement, risk assessment, safeguarding, recovery-oriented care, and the management of complex legal frameworks relating to mental health, capacity, and consent.

4.5.5 Mental health nurses work in inpatient, community, crisis, and forensic settings. The standards by which their practice is judged reflect the particular legal and ethical demands of mental health care, rather than the delivery of physical healthcare alone.

4.5.6 On the register, these practitioners are recorded as Registered Nurse (Mental Health).

Learning disability nursing

4.5.7 Learning disability nursing is a separate field dedicated to supporting people with learning disabilities. The emphasis is on promoting health, independence, inclusion, and quality of life, frequently in community-based settings rather than acute hospitals.

4.5.8 Training and practice focus on communication, behavioural support, advocacy, safeguarding, and addressing health inequalities. Learning disability nurses often play a coordinating role, ensuring that individuals can access services and that reasonable adjustments are made to meet their needs.

4.5.9 On the register, these practitioners are recorded as Registered Nurse (Learning Disabilities).

Children's nursing

4.5.10 Children's nursing is the field concerned with the physical healthcare of infants, children, and young people. It includes neonatal care, acute paediatrics, community children's nursing, and specialist paediatric services.

4.5.11 Children's nurses are trained in child-specific physiology, development, safeguarding, and family-centred care. The legal and ethical context of practice differs materially from adult nursing, particularly in relation to consent, parental responsibility, and safeguarding duties.

4.5.12 On the register, these practitioners are recorded as Registered Nurse (Children).

Midwifery

4.5.13 Midwifery is regulated by the NMC but is a distinct profession rather than a branch of nursing. Midwives provide care to women and babies during pregnancy, labour, birth, and the postnatal period, and have a clearly defined scope of autonomous practice.

4.5.14 Midwifery has its own education standards, proficiencies, and protected title. While some individuals hold both nursing and midwifery registration, midwifery registration is distinct.

4.5.15 On the register, these practitioners are recorded as Midwife.

Nursing associates

4.5.16 Nursing associates are a separately regulated role, introduced to support the nursing workforce and to bridge the gap between healthcare support workers and registered nurses. They are subject to distinct professional standards.

4.5.17 Nursing associates are not entered into one of the four nursing fields. Their scope of practice, level of autonomy, and educational preparation are distinct, and they must practise within the limits of their role.

4.5.18 On the register, these practitioners are recorded as Nursing Associate.

5 Scope of practice

5.1 Some practitioners hold registration in more than one part of the register, for example in both adult and mental health nursing, or as both a nurse and a midwife. In such cases, the registrant is entitled to use each protected title corresponding to their registration and is expected to maintain competence within each field.

5.2 Where a registrant holds only a single field of registration, they are not considered entitled to practise outside that field simply by virtue of being a registered nurse. This distinction is frequently central to disputes about scope of practice, employer expectations, and allegations of lack of competence.

6 Touchpoints of regulatory engagement

6.1 Most registrants will have limited direct interaction with the NMC over the course of their career. The common points at which regulatory engagement becomes direct and consequential can be outlined thus:

Entry (or return) to the register

6.1.1 This includes initial registration, admission of internationally qualified applicants, and restoration following removal or lapse. These decisions determine whether an individual is legally entitled to practise under the protected professional titles and therefore engage the NMC's public protection function at its earliest point.

6.1.2 Registration is the legal gateway to authorised practice and the basis on which the public can assume a minimum level of competence, integrity and accountability.

6.1.3 Entry (or re-entry) to the register is not simply an administrative exercise. The registration process requires the NMC to be satisfied that an applicant meets threshold requirements. The NMC's function is therefore protective. The public interest does not engage only when something goes wrong in practice, but persists from the moment the public is exposed to risk through professional practice. Nurses, midwives and nursing associates interact daily with the public in circumstances of the utmost vulnerability, have access to controlled medications, are required to make clinical decisions, are privy to sensitive information, and exercise positions of trust. Their actions and decisions are capable of fatal and life-changing consequence. The statutory scheme mandates that access to such an important position of responsibility be granted only to those who demonstrably meet baseline standards.

6.1.4 The protective obligation manifests in three ways:

6.1.4.1 Threshold suitability. The NMC must be satisfied that the applicant meets the requirements of education and training and any other prerequisites, including those relating to health and character. Threshold decisions can become contested where there is previous misconduct, adverse health history, adverse findings by another regulator, or criminal history.

6.1.4.2 Lawful practice. Registration is more than an endorsement of competence; it confers a legal entitlement. That is why removal from the register has immediate practical effect. It deprives a person of the legal ability to practise in the protected roles. This is true whether removal occurs by disciplinary sanction, by lapse, or by failure to revalidate.

6.1.4.3 Continuing accountability. Registration is not a one-time affair. It is a continuing status subject to continuing standards. Once a practitioner is registered, they remain accountable to the NMC for the duration of that registration, wherever and however they practise.

6.1.5 Registration decisions are capable of challenge, and the scheme provides routes of appeal and oversight in particular contexts. The broader legal point is that these are public law decisions; decisions taken under statutory power with significant consequences. They must therefore be taken lawfully, fairly and rationally.

6.1.6 Registration also interacts with other statutory schemes, particularly criminal records disclosure and safeguarding regimes. Disclosure and Barring Service (DBS) information may affect both the NMC's assessment of suitability and an employer's ability to deploy an individual in regulated activity. The DBS regime contains statutory duties to refer information in defined circumstances. The existence of these duties, and the consequences of DBS barring decisions, can be practically decisive for a registrant's ability to work with vulnerable groups, even where the NMC has not taken action or has not yet concluded action. The statutory regimes are distinct, but the same facts often engage both.

Revalidation

6.1.7 Registration is a continuing status which must be maintained through regular revalidation. Revalidation is one of the principal points at which the NMC's regulatory relationship with registrants is experienced by the profession as a whole.

6.1.8 Revalidation requires registrants, at prescribed intervals, to demonstrate continued engagement with practice and with professional standards. It typically includes requirements relating to practice hours, continuing professional development (CPD), reflective accounts, professional discussion and confirmation. Conceptually, revalidation is not a re-examination of competence, but a supervised review of reflection, accountability, continued learning and engagement with standards.

6.1.9 Failure to revalidate has automatic consequences. If a registrant does not successfully revalidate, they are removed from the register. The removal is regulatory rather than disciplinary, but it has the same practical effect: the registrant may not lawfully practise in the protected roles.

Raising concerns

6.1.10 Concerns may be referred by employers, colleagues, service users, other regulators or the police. Registrants may also (and are in certain circumstances required to) self-refer. The NMC's guidance reflects an expectation that employers will ordinarily act first to address concerns about practice, unless the risk is so serious that immediate regulatory action is required. Referrals should explain the steps taken locally and why they were insufficient. Members of the public are similarly encouraged to raise concerns with employers in the first instance where appropriate. This is not a jurisdictional rule. It is a practical and policy approach to proportionality and regulatory resource.

6.1.11 The nature of concerns capable of engaging the regulator is wide. The critical question is not whether the conduct occurred in the workplace, but whether it engages one or more statutory grounds and, if so, whether it raises an issue of fitness to practise.

Interim action

6.1.12 In cases where there is an alleged immediate risk to public safety or to public confidence, the NMC may seek interim conditions of practice or interim suspension while an investigation or hearing is ongoing. Interim orders are protective rather than punitive. Their justification lies in risk management rather than findings of misconduct.

The fitness to practise (FTP) process

6.1.13 Once concerns pass the statutory threshold, the registrant may become subject to investigation and, in appropriate cases, formal adjudication. This is the point at which regulatory engagement becomes overtly legal.

6.1.14 Allegations are formulated by reference to statutory grounds, evidence is gathered and tested, and the registrant's fitness to practise is assessed by an independent tribunal. The detail of the FTP process forms the majority of the content of this book.

Review and restoration

6.1.15 Final orders may impose conditions, suspend registration or remove a registrant from the register entirely. Many orders are subject to review at defined intervals, and all orders short of strike-off are reviewed before expiration.

6.1.16 A registrant's ability to return to unrestricted practice commonly depends on evidence of insight, remediation and effective management of risk.

6.2 These touchstones frequently coincide with other statutory or legal processes arising from the same underlying events. Safeguarding regimes may be engaged where concerns relate to abuse or neglect, including section 42 Care Act enquiries. The DBS regime may be engaged where a person is removed from regulated activity because they have caused harm or pose a risk of harm. Coronial proceedings may arise where a death has occurred. Civil proceedings may also be pursued, including claims in negligence arising out of alleged clinical failings. Criminal investigations or prosecutions may proceed in parallel, and the outcome of criminal proceedings may itself constitute a statutory ground for regulatory action. Employer processes frequently run alongside all of these, applying different tests and serving different purposes.

6.3 Parallel processes are common, given that serious incidents seldom trigger only one protective regime. There is often pressure to await the outcome of other proceedings before progressing with regulatory proceedings. Often that is appropriate. Sometimes it is not. The NMC's protective function can require action even where other processes are ongoing, particularly where risk is immediate. Interim orders are often the mechanism used to address risk pending the conclusion of other proceedings.

6.4 In practice, one of the most important skills for lawyers undertaking NMC work is the ability to disentangle overlapping regimes and parallel proceedings. This requires identifying which questions properly belong to which process, managing the flow of evidence and disclosure between them, and ensuring that engagement with one process does not prejudice the investigation, process or a registrant's position in another.

6.5 Material generated in one forum, including employer investigations, safeguarding enquiries, inquests, civil proceedings or criminal cases, may later be relied upon in fitness to practise proceedings. Such material must be approached with careful attention to relevance, fairness and statutory purpose, recognising that findings made for one legal purpose are not determinative of regulatory outcomes.

7 Relationship with NHS bodies

7.1 Many referrals originate from NHS employers, and the NMC's work frequently intersects with NHS governance. The relationship is close in practice but distinct in law.

7.2 Employer disciplinary and capability processes are directed at employment. Their purpose is to manage workforce standards, protect patients within the employer's service, address contractual obligations, and employer reputation. Employers can impose conditions of employment, redeploy staff, suspend staff, or dismiss staff. These powers are managerial. They are not regulatory.

7.3 FTP proceedings are directed at public-facing values and registration. Their purpose is to determine whether a message needs to be sent to the public and profession as a whole, and whether a registrant remains fit to practise and therefore entitled to remain on the register (restricted or otherwise).

7.4 The NMC itself recognises that employers are often best placed to act first in relation to practice concerns and expects employers to provide details of the steps taken to address concerns before referral, unless the risk is so serious that immediate regulatory action is required. That approach is rooted in proportionality and in the practical reality that employers can intervene quickly and can directly manage risk in the workplace.

7.5 The overlap between employer processes and regulation, however, generates recurrent forensic issues. Registrants and witnesses alike often demonstrate a temptation to treat NMC proceedings as an appeal against an employer's decision. Such an approach is erroneous. The NMC does not determine whether an employer acted fairly or whether dismissal was lawful. Those are employment law questions. The NMC determines, based upon its own independent assessment of the facts, whether the registrant's fitness to practise is impaired.

8 Procedural rules

8.1 The 2001 Order establishes the statutory foundation for the NMC's regulatory functions, but those functions are given procedural effect through a series of distinct statutory instruments, each directed to a specific regulatory task.

8.2 Registration, readmission and registration appeals are governed separately by the *Nursing and Midwifery Council (Education, Registration and Registration Appeals) Rules 2004* (the Registration rules). These rules regulate entry to the register, renewal, lapse, readmission and appeals against registration decisions. Education and training are regulated through the same rules, together with standards issued by the NMC under the 2001 Order.

8.3 FTP proceedings are governed principally by the *Nursing and Midwifery Council (Fitness to Practise) Rules 2004* (the FTP rules). The FTP rules regulate the investigation and adjudication of allegations, the imposition of interim measures, the conduct of substantive hearings, the review of orders and the disposal of cases. Proceedings under the FTP rules are concerned with past conduct only insofar as it informs the present question of impairment and the need for protective regulatory intervention. Adjudication under the FTP rules is carried out by one of two Practise Committees.[2]

8.3.1 The Investigating Committee exercises a gatekeeping role at the pre-hearing stage, determining whether

2 Article 3(9), *Nursing and Midwifery Order 2001*

allegations should be referred for adjudication or disposed of by other statutory means.

8.3.2 The Fitness to Practise Committee determines whether a registrant's fitness to practise is impaired by reason of any of the grounds set out in Article 22 of the 2001 Order. The Fitness to Practise Committee was previously divided between, but now sits as a combination of:[3]

8.3.2.1 The Conduct and Competence Committee, panels of which determine cases where impairment is alleged by reason of misconduct, lack of competence, conviction or caution, or adverse determinations by other regulators.

8.3.2.2 The Health Committee, panels of which which have exclusive jurisdiction where impairment is alleged by reason of physical or mental health.

8.4 The makeup and rules of appointment to those committees are governed by the *Nursing and Midwifery Council (Practice Committees) (Constitution) Rules 2008* (the Constitution rules).

9 Supervisory jurisdiction and appeals

9.1 The High Court

9.1.1 The interim order powers of the NMC are capped to the extent that interim orders may be made for a maximum duration of 18 months. Extensions are increasingly commonplace, but extension beyond 18

---

3 *Nursing and Midwifery (Amendment) Order* 2017

months is the preserve of the High Court. The NMC may apply to the High Court under Article 31 of the 2001 Order to extend an interim order by no more than 12 months; though subsequent extension requests can be made at the expiry of any such extension(s).

9.1.2 Final FTP decisions are also subject to oversight. The 2001 Order provides for appeals against specified decisions and orders. The route is again to the High Court; a statutory appeal rather than judicial review. The precise scope of the appeal depends on the decision being challenged.

9.1.3 Such appeals are not rehearings. The High Court's role is supervisory in character. It is concerned with whether the tribunal has erred in law, acted unfairly, reached an irrational conclusion, failed to take account of relevant matters, taken account of irrelevant matters, or imposed a sanction that is wrong in the sense recognised by professional discipline appeals. The court is not ordinarily concerned to reweigh evidence merely because it might have reached a different conclusion.

9.1.4 This reflects a broader jurisprudential balance unfamiliar to many practitioners in different areas of law. Panels are specialist tribunals tasked with applying professional standards and evaluating risk and trust. Though the High Court has a supervisory role to ensure legality, fairness, rationality, and proper reasoning, particular deference is paid to the 'specialist' decisions of FTP panels; the High Court seldom assumes the role of primary decision-maker.

9.1.5 Judicial review remains available in relation to decisions for which there is no adequate alternative remedy by statutory appeal, including some interim and procedural decisions. Judicial review is not a route for rearguing merits. It is a route for challenging legality, fairness and rationality.

9.2 The Professional Standards Authority

9.2.1 Though the NMC has no power to appeal decisions of its own panels, the NMC is subject to oversight by the Professional Standards Authority (PSA). The PSA is the oversight body for the healthcare regulators. It reviews final FTP decisions and may refer cases to the High Court where it considers that a decision is insufficient for the protection of the public. The power to do so derives from section 29 of the *National Health Service Reform and Health Care Professions Act 2002.*

9.2.2 The statutory language of section 29 is broad and is directed at the sufficiency of decisions for public protection. The PSA explains that it reviews every final decision and may refer cases where it considers that the decision is insufficient for public protection, and that this may include appealing against sanction, a finding, or a lack of a finding (including a decision not to find impairment). It is a public interest mechanism aimed at preventing undue leniency and maintaining consistency and confidence across the regulatory landscape.

9.2.3 The existence of PSA oversight has a practical effect on the conduct of NMC litigation. It encourages careful and explicit reasoning by panels, particularly on impairment and sanction. It also makes plain that a case does not end simply because the NMC and registrant reconcile themselves with an outcome. Public interest considerations, represented through PSA oversight, remain engaged.

9.2.4 The PSA's section 29 mechanism also reflects a deeper point about professional regulation which practitioners new to the area must bear in mind. The system is not designed solely to do justice between the regulator and the registrant. It is designed to protect the public. PSA referrals are an expression of that design, and they operate as a safeguard where a regulator's tribunal is perceived to have under-achieved the statutory objectives. Where an outcome appears too good to be true for a particular registrant, it is often because the wider public interest has not been adequately reflected in the tribunal's evaluative judgement, leaving the decision vulnerable to correction on appeal by the PSA.

9.3 Fitness to practise jurisprudence does not develop in isolation within a single regulatory scheme. The courts, particularly the Administrative Court, consider appeals arising from multiple statutory regimes, including those governing doctors, nurses, dentists, pharmacists and other professionals. As a result, leading authorities of general application on misconduct, impairment, sanction, procedural fairness and proportionality frequently originate from different regulatory contexts.

9.4 Some caution is required when transposing authority across regulatory schemes, particularly where relevant authority arises outside of closely comparable healthcare regulatory schemes; "each regulatory scheme, for solicitors, for doctors, for barristers, and so on, must be construed and applied on its own terms. Great care must always be taken when seeking to apply an authority under one scheme to [a case] under a different scheme. Regulation of the professions is established under a series of discrete statutory codes; principles developed in one scheme may say little that informs the approach required in a different scheme."[4] The weight to be given to public confidence, the availability of particular sanctions, review mechanisms, and the framing of statutory grounds may differ materially. Authority from another regulator is therefore persuasive, often determinative at the level of principle, but it must always be tested against the specific language and architecture of the Nursing and Midwifery Order 2001 and the NMC rules.

10 The limits of regulatory power

10.1 The NMC's powers are significant, but not unlimited. The NMC cannot resolve employment disputes, award compensation, or determine civil liability. It cannot intervene outside statutory grounds, and it cannot lawfully pursue matters that fall outside its jurisdiction.

10.2 Understanding those limits is essential in practice, because much of the anxiety and frustration experienced by participants in NMC proceedings stems from a disparity between what they believe the NMC should and what it is legally empowered to do.

10.3 Complainants frequently wish the NMC to investigate systemic failings of NHS trusts or hospitals, poor staffing, or workplace culture. FTP proceedings cannot be used as proxies for the other remedies. Those may be serious matters, but they do not sit neatly within the NMC's jurisdiction unless they reflect the work of a single regulated person. They may be matters for employer governance, for commissioners, for NHS England,

4 *Beckwith v Solicitors Regulation Authority* [2020] EWHC 3231, at [19]

for the Care Quality Commission, or for safeguarding bodies. They are, however, largely outwith the NMC's remit; the fitness to practise of each individual on the register.

10.4 Similarly, registrants frequently wish the NMC to vindicate them against unfair treatment by an employer. The NMC cannot do so. Employment disputes have their own statutory and contractual mechanisms. Registrants rarely arrive at FTP proceedings in a vacuum. For many, the FTP process is the final stage in a long and bruising sequence of events: internal disciplinary proceedings, HR grievances, safeguarding investigations, suspensions, capability processes and, not uncommonly, dismissal. By the time of the FTP hearing, the registrant may have spent years contesting allegations across multiple forums, with a substantial documentary trail and a strong sense of personal injustice. That history is often emotionally weighty and, from the registrant's perspective, central to their narrative. For the practitioner, however, a clear distinction must be maintained. Much of what feels most important to a registrant may be of limited or no relevance to the statutory questions the panel must answer. Part of effective representation lies in acknowledging the significance of that history, while rigorously identifying what genuinely advances the issues of fact, impairment and sanction; ensuring that peripheral grievances do not obscure the tribunal's focused evaluative task.

10.5 The legal and practical discipline required in NMC proceedings is therefore one of separation and connection: separating distinct statutory questions and processes, while recognising the ways in which evidence, risk and outcomes can interact across regimes. Each must be understood on its own terms.

CHAPTER TWO

NMC STANDARDS

11 **Setting expectations**

11.1 The statutory framework set out in the preceding chapter manifests in the standards set by the NMC, which describe what nurses, midwives and nursing associates are expected to do, and how they are expected to behave, throughout their professional lives.

11.2 The standards are not confined in relevance to FTP proceedings. They inform decisions about entry to the register, underpin the revalidation process, and provide the reference point against which conduct, competence and professional judgement are assessed whenever concerns arise. Forming a constant thread running through a registrant's career, understanding the standards is essential to understanding how regulatory decisions are made and how professional practice is evaluated.

12 **The Code: Professional Standards**

12.1 "*The Code: Professional standards of practice and behaviour for nurses, midwives and nursing associates*", effective from 10 October 2018,[5] is the NMC's primary statement of the professional standards expected of registrants, structured into four themes and 25 numbered standards. In FTP proceedings, pleaded breaches of Code standards perform three functions that matter in advocacy: they identify the professional

[5] At the time of writing, the NMC has announced an intention to revise the Code, with consultations expected to commence in July 2026

benchmark against which facts are assessed when deciding whether conduct amounts to misconduct or lack of competence; they inform the evaluative judgement on impairment; and they assist the panel in assessing seriousness and selecting a proportionate sanction by reference to public protection, public confidence, and the maintenance of standards.

12.2 What follows is an attempt at a practical guide to each of the standards as they often arise in FTP proceedings. For each, along with commentary provided by the higher courts, the emphasis is upon: what the standard requires in fitness to practise terms; typical allegation patterns; the points that tend to matter in submissions and case management; and the usual sanction dynamics.

Standard 1: Treat people as individuals and uphold their dignity

12.3 This standard is frequently pleaded as the central benchmark in cases said to involve a failure of basic professional values. In practice, Standard 1 functions as both a conduct standard (dignity, respect, compassion) and an omission standard (fundamentals of care, delay).

12.4 The higher courts have consistently upheld the suggestion that the maintenance of patient dignity is a fundamental tenet of the profession:

> The recognition and protection of human dignity is one of the core values – in truth the core value – of our society and, indeed, of all the societies which are part of the European family of nations and which have embraced the principles of the Convention. It is a core value of the common law, long pre-dating the Convention [...] The invocation of the dignity of the patient [...] is not some

> meaningless incantation designed to comfort the living or to assuage the consciences of those involved in making life and death decisions: it is a solemn affirmation of the law's and of society's recognition of our humanity and of human dignity as something fundamental.[6]

12.5 Dignity has been interpreted widely by the courts; "it is not just the sentient or self-conscious who have dignity interests protected by the law".[7] Thus, patient dignity can be infringed in circumstances where a patient is not present physically or consciously. Derogatory or racist comments made about a patient can infringe dignity even where the patient is unaware of them: "it is no answer to say, […] that the patient would not have heard the remark because they were not sentient, being the subject of the operation. The making of such a racist remark whilst the patient is on the operating table is an affront to their dignity." [8]

12.6 The common factual patterns in FTP proceedings relating to Standard 1 include: rough or dismissive treatment of patients; humiliating language or tone; failures in personal care (nutrition, hydration, hygiene, toileting, pressure care, comfort); neglect of privacy in intimate care; delay in attending basic needs; stereotyping or discriminatory assumptions; and conduct towards vulnerable people which is said to demonstrate a lack of compassion or a failure to recognise vulnerability. In staff-on-staff cases, the standard is occasionally relied upon by

---

6 *R (A, B, X and Y) v East Sussex CC and the Disability Rights Commission (No 2)* [2003] EWHC 167 (Admin), at [86]

7 *Burke, R (on the application of) v General Medical Council Rev 1* [2004] EWHC 1879 (Admin), at [58]

8 *General Medical Council & Anor v Gilbert* [2025] EWHC 802 (Admin), at [86]. At the time of writing, pending appeal

analogy where the same "dignity" language is said to describe bullying or humiliating behaviour.

12.7 From an evidential perspective, Standard 1 allegations carry a recurrent risk of vagueness. "Lacked compassion" is frequently pleaded but rarely a finding capable of being upheld on its own; panels usually expect particularisation and supporting particulars in evidence. The forensic work, therefore, begins with specificity: what precisely is said to have been done or said, to whom, when, in what setting, and with what consequence? In omission cases, chronology is central. Bundles typically contain the clinical record, observation charts, care plans, incident reports, and witness statements. The tribunal is generally assisted by submissions that identify, with precision, what was due at each stage and what evidence supports the proposition that it did not occur.

12.8 In impairment terms, Standard 1 sits on two different spectra. At one end are cases where the failing is essentially a competence or prioritisation issue, capable of remediation through learning, supervision and structured practice. At the other end are cases that appear to reveal an attitudinal disposition: contempt, deliberate cruelty, entrenched disrespect, or persistent disregard for vulnerability. The second category is more likely to engage the public component of impairment.

12.9 Sanction dynamics are correspondingly variable. One-off lapses in tone, or isolated failures in the fundamentals of care occurring in a complex or emergency context and accompanied by prompt reflection, may attract outcomes that mark the failing without removing the registrant from practice, particularly where a workable conditions package can manage any residual risk.

12.10 Patterns of neglect and humiliating behaviour are commonly treated as serious, and often lead to suspension at the least.

Given the particular vulnerability of many patients, strike-off often follows where treatment is particularly cruel. In *Ajana*,[9] for example, the High Court considered strike-off to be a proper and reasonable outcome where a midwife "repeatedly act[ed] with hostility towards women who were at times alone, vulnerable, in pain, exhausted, and no doubt desperate for kind and safe care."[10]

<u>Standard 2: Listen to people and respond to their preferences and concerns</u>

12.11 Standard 2 is frequently engaged in cases relating to communication, responsiveness, consent and shared decision-making. It is not a requirement to accede to patient preference, but a requirement to engage appropriately with preference and concern.

12.12 Common factual patterns include: failures to follow birth plans; dismissing or minimising reported symptoms; failing to explain treatment decisions; failing to reassess when concern is raised; and failing to recognise distress (including distress caused by pain, confusion, anxiety, bereavement or mental ill-health).

12.13 Evidentially, Standard 2 cases are often won on chronology and contemporaneous material. Call bell logs, observation charts, nursing notes, handover sheets, escalation documentation, incident reports and witness accounts all carry weight. Panels frequently test whether the alleged failure is genuinely one of non-response, or whether the care occurred but the patient's preferences were not documented to an acceptable standard, or the explanation was inadequate. A defence case often succeeds where it shows that the registrant assessed, acted and escalated

9 *Ajana v Nursing and Midwifery Council* [2025] EWHC 3179 (Admin)

10 *Ajana*, at [38]

appropriately but communication did not meet the ideal. A prosecuting case often succeeds where it shows repeated failure to act on concerns, avoidable delay in reassessment, or an indifference to distress that a reasonable practitioner would have addressed.

12.14 In impairment terms, Standard 2 breaches are commonly remediable. They often lend themselves to evidence of learning and changed practice, including reflection on communication, structured training, feedback, and demonstrable improvement (ossified in a lack of repetition since the index events). However, the standard can engage public impairment where the failing is repeated, involves vulnerable people, results in significant harm, or is accompanied by dishonesty about what was done. In such cases, the public interest in maintaining confidence may feature more prominently.

12.15 Sanction typically follows that analysis. Where a concern is remediable and the registrant demonstrates insight, conditions can often manage risk. Where the concern involves persistent disregard of distress, repeated non-responsiveness, or misconduct bound up with concealment or hostility, suspension becomes more likely.

12.16 The professional duty of candour guidance can be relevant where a concern relates to something having gone wrong and the allegation is not merely poor communication but a failure of openness and explanation.

Standard 3: Make sure that needs are assessed and responded to

12.17 Standard 3 is the Code's holistic assessment and wellbeing standard. It requires attention to wellbeing and changing needs during care. It is often pleaded in cases where the regulator says the registrant failed not merely to perform a task, but to recognise need and respond appropriately.

12.18 Common factual patterns include omissions in basic care and monitoring; failures to recognise deterioration; failure to address pain; failure to report safeguarding concerns; and inadequate end-of-life care. It may also engage where a registrant is said to have failed to challenge poor practice or discriminatory behaviour by others.

12.19 Evidentially, Standard 3 allegations demand a careful account of what was known, what was assessed, and what action followed. Panels often examine whether the alleged needs were documented and the extent of information conveyed on handover, whether observations and assessments were undertaken, whether care plans were implemented, and whether escalation occurred. In cases framed as failures to advocate, evidence often includes witness accounts of what was raised, what response followed, and whether the registrant used available channels to challenge or escalate.

12.20 In impairment analysis, Standard 3 cases are frequently considered remediable. Where the concern is essentially a skills and prioritisation deficit, conditions can often be crafted to target the identified risk. However, repeated omission in basic care can be characterised as a serious departure from professional standards, particularly where vulnerability is present, because the fundamentals of nursing are engaged. The tribunal's reasoning often turns on whether the registrant accepts the seriousness of omissions and can demonstrate practical learning and remediation rather than abstract regret.

12.21 Isolated omissions with strong insight and credible improvement may attract conditions or a caution depending on seriousness. Patterns of neglect, repeated failures to recognise distress or deterioration, and failures in end-of-life compassion can attract suspension, particularly where the panel cannot be satisfied that the risk is adequately managed.

12.22 Safeguarding guidance frequently becomes relevant when the case involves vulnerability, neglect or abuse risk, or failures to advocate.

Standard 4: Act in the best interests of people at all times

12.23 Standard 4 has a more explicitly legal focus than other parts of the Code. It requires balancing best interests with refusal of treatment, properly informed consent, compliance with mental capacity law and managing conscientious objection by disclosure and handover. In practice, it is often pleaded as an umbrella standard, but it has particular relevance in consent, capacity and boundary cases where a failure to prioritise the patient's interests is alleged.

12.24 Factual patterns include: proceeding without valid consent; inadequate explanation of treatment; failure to document consent; failure to respect refusal and failure to apply mental capacity principles. It can also appear in cases where a registrant is said to have put their own interests first (for example by concealing error or failing to escalate because of fear of criticism) or where the registrant has administered care while impaired by alcohol or drugs.

12.25 Evidentially, consent and capacity cases usually are record-driven. Panels look for documentation, contemporaneous records, evidence of discussion at local or MDT level, and where appropriate evidence of capacity assessments or best interests decision-making. Defence cases often turn on demonstrating that the registrant's actions were clinically justified in the particular (often emergency) circumstances, that consent was obtained and explained, and that any documentation shortfall did not equate to absence of consent.

Prosecution cases often turn on showing that consent was assumed, that refusal was overridden without lawful basis, or that capacity principles were misunderstood or ignored.

12.26 In impairment and sanction terms, these cases vary widely. Technical documentation failures may be remediable and lend themselves to conditions or a caution depending on seriousness. More serious cases, involving conscious disregard of capacity law, coercion, or repeated failures to respect refusal, can engage public confidence and lead to suspension, because they implicate fundamental respect for autonomy and lawful practice.

12.27 Sanction dynamics vary accordingly. Technical, remediable and remediated deficiencies may not warrant sanction at all. Conversely, in *Namusisi*,[11] a case involving a nurse falling asleep on duty and leaving a patient in a locked room at risk of aspiration, the High Court considered that where a breach of Standard 4 "put a vulnerable patient at risk of severe harm [and] actions were said to be deliberate, planned, wholly unacceptable and selfish. [... The] only proper sanction is one of erasure from the register."[12]

<u>Standard 5: Respect people's right to privacy and confidentiality</u>

12.28 Standard 5 is central to confidentiality cases and is increasingly engaged where data protection concerns arise. It encompasses privacy in all aspects of care; both "non-disclosure" misconduct (inappropriate sharing) and "disclosure" failures (failing to

---

11 *Professional Standards Authority v Nursing and Midwifery Council & Namusisi* [2023] EWHC 1230 (Admin)

12 *Namusisi*, at [48] – [51]

share information when necessary for safety), though the former is more common.

12.29 Common fact patterns include: accessing records without clinical justification; disclosing patient information in public areas; sharing information in messaging groups; and posting or discussing patients online. Another recurring pattern concerns failures to share necessary information with colleagues where safety requires it, sometimes pleaded as a confidentiality misunderstanding.

12.30 Evidential issues often involve access logs and technical evidence on whether a particular practitioner accessed information on shared or communal devices. The tribunal will typically focus on whether the person was identifiable, whether the disclosure was necessary, whether the registrant appreciated the confidentiality duty, and whether the conduct was careless or deliberate.

12.31 Impairment and sanction depend heavily on classification. A careless one-off disclosure, promptly acknowledged and remediated, often sits within the *Cohen* framework and may be capable of management through conditions and training. Deliberate misuse, particularly for personal motives or accompanied by concealment, is commonly characterised as an integrity issue engaging the public component of impairment. In serious cases, the tribunal may conclude that trust is so undermined that strike-off is required.

12.32 NMC social media guidance is often the most useful regulator document in digital confidentiality disputes, both because it is accessible and because it frames the NMC's expectations in modern communication contexts.

Standard 6: Always practise in line with the best available evidence

12.33 Standard 6 is principally used as a foundation for competence-type allegations, though it may also be used to frame misconduct where departures are reckless or repeated. The standard is commonly pleaded in medication error cases, infection prevention, monitoring and escalation, and in advice-giving contexts.

12.34 Panels tend to be assisted by careful identification of the relevant policy, protocol, guideline or accepted practice, and a clear demonstration of the registrant's departure from it. Defence cases commonly focus on context (availability of information, complexity of presentation, staffing pressures) and on whether the deviation was clinically justified or an honest mistake.

12.35 In impairment and sanction terms, Standard 6 is often remediable. Where the deficit is specific, training and supervised practice can be targeted. Conditions are often a proportionate disposal where risk can be managed and there is evidence of learning. Suspension becomes more likely where the deficit is broad, persistent, or accompanied by limited insight, where the panel cannot be satisfied that safe practice can be delivered.

Standard 7: Communicate clearly

12.36 Standard 7 is capable of covering almost any factual setting: communication with patients, colleagues, and the public.

12.37 Factual patterns include poor handovers, unclear instructions, failure to communicate escalation, failure to explain treatment, misunderstandings with colleagues, and failures to check comprehension. In some cases, Standard 7 is pleaded alongside record keeping, because documentation is treated as a form of communication.

12.38 Evidentially, the tribunal often looks to the consequence of the alleged communication failure. Panels are generally reluctant to impose serious sanctions for communication defects that are stylistic, though repeated patterns can still be treated as serious where they undermine safe care.

12.39 Remediation is usually straightforward: training, feedback, reflection, and demonstrable change. Conditions are frequently workable where the communication defect relates to handover or documentation. Suspension tends to arise where communication failures result in serious harm, are repeated, and appear resistant to improvement, or where the communication failure is tied to dishonesty or hostility. In *Holder*,[13] the High Court upheld a sanction of strike-off and accepted the proposition that "speaking inappropriately to colleagues in earshot of patients; shouting at office staff; [and] confronting a doctor in the presence of a patient" might each individually be sufficiently serious as to amount to misconduct.

Standard 8: Work co-operatively

12.40 Standard 8 is the Code's principal teamwork standard, concerned with safety and quality as well as collegiality.

12.41 Factual patterns include failure to share information, poor handovers, refusal to seek assistance, undermining MDT working, and workplace conflicts that affect safety. In some cases, Standard 8 is pleaded where there is alleged bullying or intimidation.

[13] *Holder v Nursing and Midwifery Council* [2017] EWHC 1565 (Admin), at [12] & [72]

12.42 The forensic hazard is over-generalisation. Panels will usually expect to know what cooperation was required in the situation and how significantly the registrant failed to reach that standard. Where the allegation is essentially that the registrant was a "difficult colleague", the tribunal is more likely to focus on whether safety, communication, and professional behaviour were actually compromised. Evidence typically includes statements from colleagues, internal HR complaints, contemporaneous emails or messages, and incident reports.

12.43 In impairment and sanction terms, many Standard 8 cases are frequently remediable. They often lend themselves to reflection and behavioural change, and conditions may be workable if the concern is about structured communication. However, where the conduct includes intimidation, refusal to cooperate in safety-critical contexts, or persistent undermining of colleagues, the tribunal may treat it as misconduct with a public confidence dimension, particularly where patient safety is affected.

12.44 Raising concerns and whistleblowing guidance becomes relevant when a registrant asserts that their non-cooperation was in truth legitimate escalation or refusal to participate in unsafe practice.

<u>Standard 9: Share your skills, knowledge and experience for the benefit of people receiving care and your colleagues</u>

12.45 Standard 9 is commonly engaged in supervision, teaching, and workplace culture cases. It is a standard that links to safe practice.

12.46 Common fact patterns include poor supervision of junior staff, refusal to support students, unconstructive behaviour towards colleagues, and inability to deal professionally with disagreements.

12.47 Evidence often turns on role, expectations and teaching style. The tribunal will commonly consider the registrant's seniority, whether they were tasked with supervision, and whether support was reasonably required. Documentary evidence of supervision arrangements, training records, and witness accounts often feature. Defence cases often rely upon workload, unclear role expectations, or isolated conflict.

12.48 In impairment and sanction terms, failures under Standard 9 are frequently remediable. Where the concern is behavioural and interpersonal, the tribunal will look for insight, acceptance of responsibility, and credible evidence of changed approach. Where the behaviour is bullying-adjacent or reflects hostility towards junior colleagues or those with protected characteristics, the case may be treated as more serious, with suspension possible particularly where the registrant occupies a role of responsibility.

Standard 10: Keep clear and accurate records relevant to your practice

12.49 Standard 10 is among the most litigated standards and one of the most sanction-sensitive, because it explicitly sets out the duty to act where someone else breaches the requirements. Its sub-paragraphs are particularly prescriptive.

12.50 Factual patterns range from incomplete notes, late entries, and sloppy documentation to deliberate falsification, fabricated observations, and concealment of error. A common pleading approach is to list multiple record keeping defects, but the tribunal's analysis usually turns on the most serious aspect: whether the record is unreliable because of dishonesty, or whether it is poor because of incompetence.

12.51 Evidentially, these cases are document-heavy and often amenable to objective proof. Audit trails, metadata, access logs, staff rotas, timing of entries, and contemporaneous other records can be decisive. Defence cases often focus on innocent explanation for lateness, context of record creation, and absence of intent to mislead. It is usually essential to separate three categories that are sometimes elided in pleadings: late entries (which may be poor practice and create risk, but are not necessarily false); inaccurate entries (which may be careless or incompetent); and false entries (which are dishonest). The classification will often drive everything that follows. A late entry that is clearly identified and is consistent with other contemporaneous material is commonly treated very differently from an entry designed to create a false picture of care, observations or escalation that did not occur.

12.52 Impairment and sanction depend on classification. Record keeping is considered essential for delivery of safe care (a fundamental tenet of the profession), and failures in record keeping are often pleaded as giving rise to serious danger of patient harm. Poor record keeping, though often remediable and addressed through training, audit, and supervision (with conditions of practice an obvious disposal where patient safety risk can be managed) nonetheless often engages the public interest and the need to declare and uphold proper standards. Sanctions vary enormously, with isolated failures resultant from identifiable stressors being unlikely to cross the misconduct threshold, to falsification and deliberate dishonesty which engage the public component of impairment and carry a substantial risk of strike-off.

12.53 Social media guidance is sometimes relevant where informal communications between colleagues are treated as "records" or where disclosure and record-keeping concerns overlap.

Standard 11: Be accountable for your decisions to delegate tasks and duties to other people

12.54 Standard 11 is a key standard in patient safety cases, though infrequently pleaded in isolation.

12.55 Factual patterns include delegation to untrained or volunteer staff and failure to supervise. In medication administration and observation contexts, unsafe delegation can often be alleged.

12.56 Evidence usually focuses upon job and role descriptions, competence documentation, supervision records, preceptorship or staged return to work plans and clinical outcome evidence. Defence cases often focus on the reasonableness of the delegation decision given what was known about the delegate's competence, and on whether supervision was in fact provided or made available.

12.57 In impairment and sanction terms, the actual or potential harm to patients plays a significant role. Standard 11 cases may be remediable where the registrant accepts the error, understands the delegation principles, and can demonstrate change. Conditions can be crafted to control delegation, supervision and review. Repeated or dramatically unsafe delegation, particularly if accompanied by lack of insight, increases the likelihood of suspension.

Standard 12: Have in place an indemnity arrangement which provides appropriate cover for any practice you take on

12.58 Standard 12 is narrow. The evidential basis for cases in which this standard is engaged is usually documentary and straightforward: whether indemnity existed, whether it was appropriate to scope of practice, and whether the registrant knew of the requirements.

12.59 In many cases, the breach is technical and remediable, particularly where indemnity was overlooked rather than deliberately avoided. However, the standard can become more serious where lack of indemnity is part of a broader picture of unsafe or unauthorised practice, or where the registrant misrepresented their cover. Lack of indemnity cover may be particularly serious where the public may have been misled. In *Briggs*,[14] for example, the argument was made of a chiropractor practising without adequate indemnity cover that "by practising as he did, he misled the public who would have thought that he was entitled to practise and that he had appropriate insurance."[15]

12.60 Impairment and sanction are therefore often driven by context. Where indemnity is promptly obtained and the registrant demonstrates understanding, circumstances may not support a suggestion of current impairment. Where the breach reflects wanton disregard of professional obligations or accompanies other misconduct, it may contribute to an adverse impairment and sanction outcome.

Standard 13: Recognise and work within the limits of your competence

12.61 Standard 13 is the central competence-limit standard in the "preserve safety" theme. It is not merely about technical ability; it is about judgement, escalation and self-management. Its sub-paragraphs require accurate observation and assessment, timely referral and asking for help where action is beyond competence. The standard is frequently pleaded where independent practice

---

[14] *Professional Standards Authority v General Chiropractic Council & Briggs* [2014] EWHC 2190 (Admin)

[15] *Briggs*, at [10]

has been unsafe or where the registrant failed to seek appropriate support.

12.62 Factual patterns include failure to recognise deterioration, failure to escalate, undertaking procedures without training or supervision, failure to refer appropriately, and unsafe practice in unfamiliar roles. It also appears in cases where fatigue, health, or personal factors are alleged to have impaired safe practice and the registrant failed to manage those risks.

12.63 Evidence often turns on establishing a pattern of practice, as isolated lapses tend to be treated as less serious than repeated errors indicative of an inability or refusal to recognise and respect limits. Panels often examine whether support was available, whether the registrant sought it, and whether escalation and referral occurred. Defence cases often focus on context, availability of senior support, and whether the registrant acted reasonably given the information available.

12.64 In impairment and sanction terms, practitioners are wise to recall that maintaining patient safety is considered a fundamental tenet of the profession, hence any failure to do so is of the utmost seriousness. If the registrant can show learning, changed practice, and credible supervision arrangements, concerns may be remediated.

12.65 In sanction terms, conditions are often appropriate where safe practice can be assured by restrictions, supervision, and training. Suspension becomes more likely where the registrant cannot demonstrate reliable improvement or where the departure from standards invokes the public interest in a declaratory sanction, for example where a registrant has deliberately practised outside the scope of supernumerary or supervised practice.[16]

Standard 14: Be open and candid with all service users, including when any mistakes or harm have taken place

12.66 Standard 14 is the Code's principal candour standard, and it is often determinative because it distinguishes between error and integrity. Medical practitioners will be well familiar with the duty of candour. It carries both an ethical dimension (honesty) and a safety dimension (documentation and escalation).

12.67 Factual patterns include failure to disclose error, minimisation or misleading explanations, failure to apologise appropriately, failure to document incidents or submit DATIX reports, and failure to escalate concerns arising from harm. Where the allegation includes dishonesty, the standard is frequently pleaded alongside record keeping and professionalism standards.

12.68 Evidence often includes incident reports, entries in clinical records, statements from patients or families, communications with colleagues, and patient notes. The key issues are usually whether the registrant knew that something had gone wrong, what was said, what was documented, and whether any concealment occurred. Panels tend to distinguish between poor communication in a difficult situation and deliberate deception.

12.69 Impairment and sanction dynamics reflect that distinction. Where the registrant accepts error, demonstrates candour and learning, and can show changed approach, the concern may be remediable. Where dishonesty is proved, public confidence

[16] See: *Fabiyi v Nursing and Midwifery Council* [2012] EWHC 1441 (Admin)

considerations are often determinative as the concern evolves from whether the registrant can practise safely, to whether they can be trusted to be open about mistakes and risks when they arise. Conditions of practice may be argued to be inadequate where the core failing is integrity rather than competence. Dishonest concealment is likely to result in strike-off.

<u>Standard 15: Always offer help if an emergency arises in your practice setting or anywhere else</u>

12.70 Standard 15 is engaged less frequently than many other standards. The standard recognises that the duty to assist is not a duty to act beyond competence or to put oneself at unreasonable risk.

12.71 Impairment and sanction will follow the seriousness of the outcome and the registrant's insight. Many cases are remediable and capable of conditions or a caution, but reckless emergency conduct causing serious harm may justify suspension and strike-off.

<u>Standard 16: Act without delay if you believe that there is a risk to patient safety or public protection</u>

12.72 Standard 16 requires raising and escalating concerns about safety or care standards including immediate escalation where asked to practise beyond role or training. It covers both raising concerns and responding to concerns.

12.73 Common fact patterns include failure to escalate unsafe staffing arrangements, ignoring colleague warnings, trivialising concerns raised by others, and retaliatory conduct against whistleblowers. It can also be pleaded where a registrant in a management role is said to have failed to protect staff who raised concerns.

12.74 Evidence is often a mixture of documentation and witness accounts: emails, incident reports, DATIX entries, meeting notes, messages, and statements. Panels generally focus on what the registrant knew, what they reasonably believed, what channels were available, and whether the response was prompt and proportionate. Defence cases often succeed where they show some escalation did occur or where the registrant took reasonable steps within their role.

12.75 In impairment and sanction terms, escalation failures can be serious because they can foster ongoing risk. Where the failure is an isolated judgement lapse, remediation is possible. Where the failure is a pattern, or where the registrant obstructed or victimised others, public confidence considerations are likely to be prominent and more restrictive sanctions become likely.

Standard 17: Raise concerns immediately if you believe a person is vulnerable or at risk and needs extra support and protection

12.76 Standard 17 is a safeguarding standard. It requires taking reasonable steps to protect those vulnerable or at risk from harm, and complying with relevant laws and policies about protecting vulnerable people and disclosure. It is most suited to cases involving alleged failure to report abuse or neglect, failure to follow safeguarding procedures, and failure to recognise vulnerability particularly in community-based care settings.

12.77 Factual patterns include non-reporting of safeguarding concerns, failure to escalate suspected abuse, failure to act on disclosures, inadequate information sharing or notes of patient interactions, and failures in safeguarding documentation. It may also arise in cases involving boundary issues and vulnerability.

12.78 Evidence often includes safeguarding referrals (or their proven absence), contemporaneous notes of disclosures, incident reports, policy documents, and witness accounts. Panels often examine whether the risk was reasonably apparent, whether the registrant understood the safeguarding obligation, and what steps were open. Defence cases may focus on competing clinical priorities and whether the registrant reasonably believed others had escalated.

12.79 Impairment and sanction dynamics frequently tend to the more restrictive end in serious safeguarding cases, particularly where the panel concludes that the registrant's failure permitted risk to continue. Where safeguarding failures are remediable and the registrant demonstrates learning, conditions can sometimes manage risk; where the failure is grave or repeated, suspension becomes feasible.

<u>Standard 18: Advise on, prescribe, supply, dispense or administer medicines within the limits of your training and competence, the law, our guidance and other relevant policies, guidance and regulations</u>

12.80 Standard 18 is framed to apply across the range of medicines activities, recognising that not all registrants prescribe. It spans competence, governance, integrity and boundaries.

12.81 Factual patterns include self-prescribing, medication errors, dose and route errors, poor controlled drug handling, inadequate documentation, unsafe storage, and in serious cases diversion and falsification of records. Cases involving prescribing for family and friends also arise, though less frequently.

12.82 Evidence often includes controlled drug logs, MAR charts, audit data, incident reports, and expert evidence where the clinical significance is disputed. Panels commonly focus on whether the error was an isolated lapse or a pattern, whether systems contributed, whether the registrant understood medicines governance, and whether there is dishonesty.

12.83 Medication errors are inherently dangerous. Many medications are stringently controlled drugs, given their propensity to do harm in the wrong circumstances or dosage. Panels tend to therefore consider medication errors anxiously. It does not follow, however, that all errors are to be treated as *equally* serious; a panel considering a medication error should consider "all the surrounding circumstances and asking how grave the [error] was. It is often the case in a medical setting that a minor mistake can have serious consequences sadly, but that does not convert negligence into gross negligence by itself."[17]

12.84 Impairment and sanction vary accordingly. Many medication errors are remediable and can be managed with conditions and supervision, provided the registrant demonstrates genuine insight and targeted learning. Repeated unsafe medicines practice, poor governance, or lack of insight can lead to suspension or beyond given the clear danger to patient safety. Where controlled drugs concerns involve dishonesty, diversion, or concealment, sanctions are often highly restrictive, because integrity and public protection are firmly engaged.

Standard 19: Be aware of, and reduce as far as possible, any potential for harm associated with your practice

12.85 Standard 19 functions as a broad risk-reduction and safety culture standard. It requires measures to reduce mistakes, near misses and harm, and mitigate harm if it occurs. It captures

[17] *Hindmarch v Nursing and Midwifery Council* [2016] EWHC 2233, at [39]

both individual practice and an awareness of systems and human factors.

12.86 Factual patterns include infection prevention failures, unsafe shortcuts, failure to adopt known safety measures, failure to learn from near misses, and failures to mitigate risks in high-pressure contexts. It is often pleaded in health cases where registrants have failed to act upon their own deteriorating health such that they have practised while unsafe to do so.

12.87 Evidentially, Standard 19 allegations benefit from clarity as to what potential harm is alleged and what measures were reasonably expected. Infection control cases, for example, will involve policy documents, training records, incident data and sometimes expert evidence. Health cases will look for demonstrable examples of deficient practice as part of a timeline of impairment or deterioration.

12.88 In impairment and sanction terms, Standard 19 can support both competence-type disposals and more serious outcomes depending on pattern and attitude. A registrant who accepts learning, engages with safety measures, and can demonstrate changed practice may prove to have remediated. A registrant who persists in unsafe shortcuts or minimises risk may attract suspension where the panel cannot be satisfied that risk is controlled.

Standard 20: Uphold the reputation of your profession at all times

12.89 Standard 20 is the core "professionalism and trust" standard. It is often pleaded in off-duty conduct and social media cases, as well as in workplace behaviour cases involving bullying, discrimination or harassment. Its sub-paragraphs include the requirement to act with honesty and integrity, treat people fairly and without discrimination, bullying or harassment, and to comply with the laws of the country of practice.

12.90 The breadth of Standard 20 also includes maintaining boundaries, role modelling professional behaviour for students and newly qualified registrants and maintaining the health needed to carry out the professional role. It is, in substance, a multi-headed standard which overlaps with many other standards. Because of the breadth of the standard, the principal forensic task is often to identify which sub-paragraph does the real work in the particular case.

12.91 The honesty and integrity requirement in Standard 20 is paramount: "to be 'honest and trustworthy and act with integrity' is a fundamental tenet of the medical profession."[18]

> In cases of actual proven dishonesty, the balance ordinarily can be expected to fall down on the side of maintaining public confidence in the profession by a severe sanction against the practitioner concerned. Indeed, that sanction will often and perfectly properly be the sanction of erasure, even in the case of a one-off instance of dishonesty.[19]

12.92 Evidentially, these cases may be document-led (criminal records, social media posts, employer documents) or witness-led (bullying or harassment). In social media cases, screenshots, platform context, audience reach and privacy settings are commonly critical. In belief-expression cases, context matters:

---

18 *Houshian v General Medical Council* [2012] EWHC 3458, at [38]

19 *Nicholas-Pillai v General Medical Council* [2009] EWHC 1048 (Admin), at [27]

what was said, to whom, in what setting, and whether it was coercive or inappropriate.

12.93 In "at all times" cases, panels should be careful to avoid treating the code as a general moral code divorced from practice. "Professional discipline, rightly, sits relatively lightly on its members outside the workplace, but it is never entirely absent where conduct in public is concerned."[20] The question is whether the conduct, viewed in context, is sufficiently serious and sufficiently connected to professional standards, public protection or public confidence to justify regulatory intervention. The proportionality exercise is fact-sensitive and will look to: the nature of the conduct, its seriousness, repetition, insight, and any continuing risk.

12.94 Impairment and sanction are fact-sensitive. Panels commonly treat serious off-duty misconduct as engaging public confidence, particularly where dishonesty, discrimination, harassment, or exploitation is proved. Analogous authority is sometimes deployed to frame the legitimacy of "at all times" professional standards and the need for a context-sensitive proportionality analysis. Sanction ranges from caution to strike-off depending on seriousness and compatibility with continued registration.

<u>Standard 21: Uphold your position as a registered nurse, midwife or nursing associate</u>

12.95 Standard 21 addresses gifts, financial probity, and the proper use of professional status. It requires refusal of all but trivial gifts, never asking for or accepting loans from those in care or close to them and honesty and integrity in financial dealings

---

20 *Ngole v University of Sheffield (HCPC intervening)* [2017] EWHC 2669 (Admin), at [175]

with those in professional relationships. It therefore captures boundary issues that are not necessarily sexual but are nevertheless exploitative or improper.

12.96 Common factual patterns include accepting significant gifts and financial exploitation. These cases often overlap with dishonesty and boundary allegations.

12.97 Evidence is often documentary: local policies on declaring gifts, receipts, bank records, messages, and witness statements from patients or families. Panels will focus on vulnerability, power imbalance, the registrant's motivation, and whether the conduct was concealed.

12.98 Impairment and sanction often engage public confidence because misuse of professional status is closely connected to trust – a fundamental tenet. Rare cases can be framed as momentary poor judgement and remediable; more frequently, particularly in cases involving exploitation, financial impropriety, or deception, serious breach of the standard is likely to be treated as incompatible with continued registration, with suspension or erasure in serious cases.

Standard 22: Fulfil all registration requirements

12.99 Standard 22 covers compliance with reasonable requests to oversee registration, prescribed hours of practice and CPD requirements. It is closely linked to revalidation in practice.

12.100 Factual patterns may include failure to meet practice hours, failure to maintain CPD, failure to respond to NMC requests, and failures in revalidation-related compliance. These cases may arise in the context of dishonesty if documentation is falsified, but many are technical or administrative.

12.101 Evidence is usually straightforward: registration records, CPD logs, correspondence with the NMC, employer records, and revalidation documentation. The tribunal's focus is often on whether the failure was inadvertent, whether it is now rectified, and whether the registrant understands the importance of ongoing professional maintenance.

12.102 Impairment and sanction are typically proportionate to risk. Many cases are remediable and may not require a restrictive outcome, unless accompanied by dishonesty or persistent disregard. Where the registrant has shown deliberate non-compliance or misrepresentation, public confidence considerations may increase the seriousness significantly.

<u>Standard 23: Cooperate with all investigations and audits</u>

12.103 Standard 23 applies to investigations and audits both against the registrant and imposes an obligation "to cooperate with internal and external investigations which related to persons other than the registrant."[21] It includes cooperating as a witness even after leaving the register. It requires disclosure to the NMC and employers of cautions, charges, conditional discharges and convictions (save for protected cautions/convictions) and disclosure to employers of restrictions or conditions imposed by the NMC or other bodies.

12.104 Common factual patterns include failure to declare convictions, failure to notify employer of restrictions, failure to provide information to the NMC, obstruction of investigations, and refusal to participate in audits. A common feature is that the failure to notify can be treated as serious in its own right,

[21] *Harford v Nursing and Midwifery Council* [2013] EWHC 696 (Admin), at [34]

because it implicates openness, integrity and the regulator's ability to manage risk.

12.105 Evidence is typically documentary: criminal records, correspondence, employer documentation, NMC communications, and investigation materials. Panels often focus on whether the registrant's failure was deliberate, reckless, or inadvertent, and whether it was motivated by concealment.

12.106 Impairment and sanction depend on that motivation. Inadvertent delays in notification may be remediable, but deliberate concealment will engage integrity and public confidence, leading to suspension or strike-off, particularly where combined with the seriousness of the underlying offence or restriction. In *Mitchell*,[22] for example, the High Court considered strike-off appropriate where a registrant had breached Standard 23, "deliberately breached her professional duty of candour and deceived her employer by failing to disclose important information which she had been required to disclose over a sustained period of some 17 months. This was serious professional misconduct which undoubtedly raised the question whether she should be allowed to remain on the register."[23]

<u>Standard 24: Respond to any complaints made against you professionally</u>

12.107 Standard 24 requires that a complaint must never affect the care provided and that complaints should be used as feedback. It is therefore concerned with retaliation, professionalism, and insight.

---

[22] *Mitchell v Nursing and Midwifery Council* [2025] EWHC 1496 (Admin)

[23] *Mitchell*, at [87]

12.108 Factual patterns include retaliatory behaviour against complainants, refusal of care, hostility towards patients who complain or the families thereof, and dismissive handling of complaints without learning. It can also appear where a registrant's communications with complainants are unprofessional or intimidating.

12.109 Evidence often includes correspondence, records of care following complaint, witness statements, and sometimes recordings or emails. Panels frequently examine whether the registrant's response was defensive in a way that undermined professionalism, and whether there is any evidence that care changed because of the complaint.

12.110 Impairment and sanction invariably turn on insight. Many complaints-handling deficits are remediable through reflection, apology and training. Retaliation, intimidation or punishment of complainants is more serious and can engage public confidence, particularly because it undermines access to feedback and patient safety culture.

Standard 25: Provide leadership to make sure people's wellbeing is protected and to improve their experiences of the health and care system

12.111 Standard 25 is framed to apply regardless of whether the registrant holds a formal leadership role. It requires identifying priorities and managing time, staff and resources effectively and dealing with risk to maintain and improve quality, putting service users. In practice, this standard often captures seniority-linked obligations: supervision, culture, safety, and resource management.

12.112 Common factual patterns often centre around ward or facility management; tolerance of unsafe practice, failure to address risks, failure to support staff development and failure to act on concerns. It may be pleaded where management decisions lead to risk, or where leaders respond inadequately to incidents.

12.113 Evidence often includes staffing rosters, incident reports, policy documents, and witness statements from staff. Panels usually calibrate expectations to role and seniority: what would be reasonable for a band 8 or ward manager may not be expected of a newly qualified registrant.

12.114 Impairment and sanction decisions can be significant where leadership failures have systemic impact or contribute to harm. Conditions restricting managerial responsibility can sometimes address deficits in leadership practice. In serious cases, particularly where leadership failures include suppression of concerns or a culture of concealment, suspension or strike-off may be necessary to protect the public and maintain confidence.

13 Proficiency standards

13.1 Proficiency standards can be invoked in misconduct cases, but more commonly feature in lack of competence matters. From a regulatory perspective, these standards perform an essential function beyond initial registration. They provide the benchmark against which concerns about competence are assessed in fitness to practise proceedings. A panel considering allegations of lack of competence must ask whether the registrant has fallen seriously below the standards reasonably expected of a registrant in their part of the register and, where relevant, their field of practice.

13.2 The NMC regulates three distinct professions, nurses, midwives and nursing associates, each of which enters practice through a different educational route, performs a different professional role, and carries different responsibilities within the healthcare system. It follows that the standards governing the professions cannot sensibly be uniform.

13.3 The obligation to prescribe standards of proficiency sits alongside the structure of the register itself. In regulatory terms, proficiency standards answer a precise question: what must a person know, understand and be able to do in order to practise safely and effectively as a member of this particular profession?

13.3.1 For nurses, the standards of proficiency are further divided by field of practice, reflecting the very different contexts in which adult, mental health, children's and learning disability nurses work. Although there is a shared professional foundation, the risks, clinical judgements, communication demands and safeguarding responsibilities vary markedly between fields. The standards therefore articulate a common core of professional capability, supplemented by field-specific expectations.

13.3.2 Midwifery standards of proficiency are distinct again. They are shaped by the midwife's autonomous role, continuity of care responsibilities, and the unique ethical and clinical dimensions of pregnancy, childbirth and the postnatal period. The standards reflect the reality that midwives are frequently the lead professionals for women and babies, making independent clinical decisions in circumstances that can evolve and deteriorate rapidly. The emphasis within the standards on partnership with women, informed choice, and advocacy integral to the scope of midwifery practice.

13.3.3 Nursing associates sit within a different regulatory and professional space. Their standards of proficiency are calibrated to a role that supports registered nurses and works under delegation, while still requiring accountability for their own practice. The standards reflect this balance. They define a distinct role with defined limits, capabilities and responsibilities. This distinction is critical both for public protection and for fairness to registrants. It makes clear what is, and is not, expected of a nursing associate, and guards against the inappropriate imposition of expectations that properly belong to another profession.

13.4 The standards of proficiency have an ongoing relevance throughout a registrant's career. They underpin education programmes, inform supervision and preceptorship, and shape the expectations against which CPD and revalidation are understood. Although they are framed as entry-level standards, they articulate the baseline from which professional growth is expected to develop.

13.5 For practitioners and panels alike, it is important to resist any temptation to treat the standards of proficiency as interchangeable across professions, or as generic statements of good practice. Their strength lies precisely in their specificity. In a system concerned above all with public protection and fairness, differentiation between roles is not merely appropriate, but essential.

CHAPTER THREE

REGISTRATION AND APPEAL

14 Introduction

14.1 Registration is the formal gateway by which an individual enters the jurisdiction of the NMC, becomes entitled to use a protected professional title, and is brought within the scope of the Code. It is the regulator's primary quality-control mechanism.

14.2 Decisions at this stage are prospective. The question is not whether the applicant has ever fallen below standards, but whether, at the date of decision, she meets the statutory and evidential requirements for admission and is suitable to practise safely and effectively.

15 Statutory and procedural framework

15.1 The power to admit individuals to the register derives from the Nursing and Midwifery Order 2001. The NMC is required to establish standards of proficiency for admission to each part of the register.

15.2 The procedural framework for registration and registration appeals is contained in the Nursing and Midwifery Council (Education, Registration and Registration Appeals) Rules 2004 (the Registration rules).

16 The Registrar's assessment

16.1 Applications for registration are determined administratively by the Registrar. The Registrar's function is not discretionary in the colloquial sense. It is a structured evaluative exercise constrained by the rules and the standards of proficiency. Where the evidential requirements are met, registration should follow. Where they are not, the application must be refused with reasons. A refusal is not a finding of misconduct or blame.

16.2 An application must comply with formal requirements of the Registration rules, including submission in the prescribed form, signature, payment of the fee,[24] and a declaration of good health and good character.[25] The applicant must provide evidence of qualification in accordance with Registration rule 5(2)(a), together with any further documents or information the Registrar may reasonably require to determine the application.[26] This may include evidence of indemnity cover,[27] and evidence of English language competence.[28]

16.3 Declarations of good health and good character must be supported by independent confirmation.[29] The precise requirements of confirmation depend on how recently the applicant has trained or practised. Where an application is made on qualification or within six months, confirmation from the senior person responsible for the approved education

---

[24] Registration rule 5.1 (initial applications); Registration rule 15 (readmission applications)

[25] Registration rule 5.1(a)

[26] Registration rule 5(2)(b)

[27] Registration rule 5(2)(aa)

[28] Registration rule 5(2)(ab)

[29] Registration rule 6(1)

programme is sufficient.[30] Where there has been a delay after qualification, or where the applicant seeks readmission without completing a return-to-practice programme, additional assurance is required from a registrant in the relevant part of the register who has known the applicant for at least a year and had recent contact.[31] Those applying for readmission may have to provide up to three references including from their most recent period of employment.[32]

16.4 For alternative routes to registration, including nursing associates and overseas applicants, character may be confirmed by an overseas licensing body where one exists, or by written evidence sufficient to satisfy the Registrar.[33]

16.5 In assessing health, the Registrar must have regard to the declaration provided by the applicant, any supporting documentation and any other information that they consider relevant.[34]

16.6 In assessing character, the Registrar must have regard to the applicant's declaration, any criminal convictions or cautions, determinations by other regulators, and any other matters appearing relevant.[35]

30 Registration rule 6(1)(a)

31 Registration rule 6(1)(b)-(c)

32 Registration rule 15(3)

33 Registration rule 6(1)(e)

34 Registration rule 6(5)

35 Registration rule 6(6)

17 Refusal

17.1 Applications may be refused for a number of reasons including: evidential insufficiency; health or character concerns (typically arising from convictions or adverse regulatory determinations); and failure to meet the English language requirement.

17.2 Where an application is refused, the Registrar must issue a written decision letter setting out the reasons and the right of appeal. Reasons should be sufficiently specific to allow the applicant to identify what evidence is missing or what concerns remain outstanding. Where reasons are unclear or generic, clarification should be sought promptly. Service may be effected electronically or by post.[36]

17.3 The appeal period is 28 days, commencing on the date of the decision letter.[37]

18 Nature and scope of registration appeals

18.1 Registration appeals are not a vehicle for relitigating historic allegations or for challenging prior disciplinary findings made elsewhere. A registration appeal is distinct from an application for restoration following strike-off.

18.2 Appeals are determined by an appeal panel.[38] The appeal panel will consider afresh whether the applicant meets the statutory and evidential requirements for entry and may substitute its own evaluative judgement for that of the Registrar.

---

[36] Registration rule 19

[37] Registration rule 20(a)

[38] Registration rule 25

18.3 Formally, the appellant must lodge a notice of appeal,[39] including the grounds of appeal and the documents relied upon. A hearing may be requested by the applicant,[40] or listed at the discretion of the NMC.[41] The appeal panel may convene a preliminary meeting where it would assist the discharging of its functions,[42] for example to determine questions of admissibility of evidence.

18.4 **Appeal hearings**

18.5 A registration appeal may be determined without an oral hearing where the appellant does not seek to attend, and the issues can properly be resolved on the papers alone. [43] An oral hearing will be listed where requested by a party or where the NMC considers it desirable.

18.6 Hearings may take place in person or remotely.[44] The appellant may be represented by a lawyer or any other person.[45] Attendance by the appellant is not compulsory, even where a hearing is convened, but is usually advantageous in providing the opportunity to give oral evidence, respond to questions from the panel, and address any outstanding concerns directly. Where an appellant does not attend, the panel may nevertheless

---

39 Registration rule 21

40 Registration rule 22(1)(a)

41 Registration rule 22(1)(b)

42 Registration rule 26

43 Registration rule 27(1)

44 Registration rule 2ZA

45 Registration rule 24(4)

proceed if satisfied that all reasonable steps have been taken to give notice of the hearing taking place.[46]

18.7 An appeal is heard by a panel of three, comprising a chair, a registrant member from the relevant part of the register, and a lay member.[47] The Panel is supported by an independent legal assessor, who advises on points of law but takes no part in decision-making, and a hearings coordinator, who manages procedure and records the determination. The NMC is represented by a case presenter who advocates for the Registrar's refusal. Both parties rely on a pre-prepared bundle containing the application, the decision letter, and any additional evidence to be relied upon.

18.8 Hearings are held in public unless the panel is satisfied that exclusion of the public is required in the interests of justice or for the protection of private life, including that of the appellant, witnesses, patients or clients.[48] Unusually, that presumption does not apply where the hearing is conducted by audio or video conferencing.[49]

Evidence

18.9 Evidence is generally governed by the rules of admissibility applicable in civil proceedings,[50] subject to the appeal panel's

[46] Registration rule 29

[47] Registration rule 25(3)

[48] Registration rule 30(1)

[49] Registration rule 30(1)(a)

[50] Registration rule 31(1)

limited power to admit otherwise inadmissible evidence where necessary to protect members of the public.[51]

18.10 The panel may require witnesses (other than the appellant) to attend and give evidence or produce documents.[52] Evidence is ordinarily given on oath or affirmation[53].

18.11 As in substantive fitness to practise proceedings, a certified certificate of conviction shall serve as conclusive proof of the conviction and the findings of fact upon which it was based.[54]

18.12 The panel may permit either party to rely on grounds or evidence not presented to the Registrar where it is just and reasonable to do so.[55] There is no prohibition on introducing new material at appeal, though applicants should be prepared to explain why it was not provided earlier. The central question remains whether, on the material now before the panel, the statutory and evidential requirements for admission are satisfied.

Order of proceedings

18.13 At the outset of the hearing, the chair will explain the order of proceedings proposed. While the precise structure may vary at the panel's discretion,[56] the rules prescribe a familiar sequence.

---

[51] Registration rule 31(3)

[52] Registration rule 31(4)

[53] Registration rule 31(7)

[54] Registration rule 31(6)

[55] Registration rule 31(5)

[56] Registration rule 30(3)

18.14 The appellant presents first,[57] calling any witnesses (including where the appellant intends to give evidence), who may be cross-examined by the case presenter,[58] then re-examined.[59]

18.15 The case presenter then advances the case in support of the decision appealed against,[60] and calls any witnesses who are again subject to cross-examination and re-examination.[61]

18.16 Closing submissions follow in reverse order, with the case presenter addressing the panel first and the appellant second.[62]

19 Outcomes

19.1 The appeal panel must notify the appellant of its decision in writing and give reasons for that decision.[63] The determination must also inform the appellant of the right of onward appeal to the county court, or in Scotland the sheriff, under Article 37 of the Nursing and Midwifery Order 2001. Such an appeal is confined to errors of law or principle rather than disagreement with the panel's evaluative judgement.

19.2 Where an appeal is unsuccessful, the refusal does not bar future applications. The applicant may submit a fresh registration application once the deficiencies identified by the Registrar or Appeal Panel have been remedied. Unlike restoration cases, there is no statutory restriction equivalent to Article 33(9)

---

[57] Registration rule 30(3)(a)

[58] Registration rule 30(3)(b)

[59] Registration rule 30(3)(b)

[60] Registration rule 30(3)(c)

[61] Registration rule 30(3)(d)

[62] Registration rule 30(3)(e) – (f)

[63] Registration rule 32

preventing further applications within a defined period. In practice, however, repeat applications unsupported by materially different evidence are unlikely to succeed.

CHAPTER FOUR

THE FTP PROCESS (OVERVIEW)

20 Conceptually

20.1 Fitness to practise (FTP) proceedings are a distinct form of statutory adjudication, governed by subordinate legislation, most obviously the Nursing and Midwifery Council (Fitness to Practise) Rules 2004 (the FTP rules).[64]

20.2 The purpose of the FTP regime is protective, not punitive. It exists to achieve the overarching objectives of Article 3(4)(a) of the 2001 Order;[65] to safeguard patients and the public, to maintain confidence in the professions regulated by the NMC, and to uphold proper professional standards. Those objectives shape every stage of the process: the framing of allegations, the assessment of evidence, the evaluation of impairment, and the selection of outcome.

20.3 FTP proceedings are therefore neither criminal prosecutions nor ordinary civil claims, and attempts to treat them as either will usually lead practitioners into error. Although the Supreme Court has historically considered disciplinary proceedings to "fall on the civil side of the line,"[66] in *R (W80) v Director*

---

64 SI 2004/1761

65 *Nursing and Midwifery Order 2001*, SI 2002/253

66 *Coke-Wallis, R (On the Application of) v Institute of Chartered Accountants in England and Wales* [2011] UKSC 1, at [24]

General of the Independent Office for Police Conduct,[67] the Supreme Court endorsed the criticism of Flaux LJ that "seeking to categorise misconduct proceedings as either criminal or civil in nature is not a profitable exercise and misconduct proceedings are essentially sui generis." Elsewhere, the courts have observed that:

> "In FTP proceedings the FPP is concerned to protect the public for the future and not to determine the rights and obligations of the parties in the same way as in a civil action. This introduces a further public interest which is not present in the ordinary civil suit."[68]

> "This is not "ordinary" civil litigation. These are proceedings conducted in the public interest and with the object of protecting the public."[69]

20.4 The unique nature of professional discipline proceedings explains several features which can be disorientating to those new to the area: the standard of proof is the civil standard; panels enjoy a broader discretion in relation to admissibility of evidence than before the courts; panels may request investigations and further evidence; and panels are bound to ensure that registrants are not "under-charged" and that the allegations reflect accurately the gravamen of the conduct alleged such that they may refuse applications to offer no evidence.

---

67 [2020] UKSC 24

68 *Meadow v General Medical Council* [2006] EWCA Civ 1390, at [33]

69 *Professional Standards Authority v General Medical Council and Zafar* [2020] EWHC 846 (Admin), at [77]

21 Where FTP sits

21.1 FTP is the legal mechanism by which the NMC determines whether a registrant should remain on the register, and on what terms. It is not synonymous with competence, though many registrants approach the process under that misapprehension. Many cases turn on conduct, integrity, health, or criminal matters rather than clinical skill. A registrant may be technically competent (even excellent) yet unfit to practise if their behaviour undermines trust, safeguarding, or public confidence.

21.2 The defining feature of the FTP regime is its forward-looking and evaluative character. The tribunal does not ask simply whether misconduct or other failings occurred in the past. Its task is to decide, in the present tense, whether the registrant's fitness to practise is impaired and, if so, what regulatory response (if any) is required to meet the statutory objectives. Past events matter, but primarily as evidence: evidence of current risk, of attitudinal failings, and of whether public confidence would be undermined if the conduct were not properly marked by a regulatory outcome.

22 The structure of decision-making at the final hearing

22.1 All final hearings follow the same sequence,[70] unless the panel determines to merge or separate stages:[71]

[70] FTP rule 24

[71] FTP rule 24(1)

The preliminary Stage

22.1.1 The panel resolves procedural and legal issues, including proceeding in absence and admissibility of evidence before the substantive hearing commences.

Stage 1

22.1.2 Findings of fact are made after hearing the evidence and submissions.

22.1.3 The tribunal determines whether any facts found proved meet one or more statutory grounds under Article 22 of the Nursing and Midwifery Order 2001.

Stage 2

22.1.4 If one or more of the statutory grounds are made out, the tribunal determines whether the registrant's fitness to practise is currently impaired.

Stage 3

22.1.5 If impairment is found, the tribunal determines what sanction, if any, is necessary to meet the statutory objectives.

22.1.6 Where conditions of practice, suspension or strike off are ordered, the Panel will consider the imposition of an interim order restricting practice during the appeal period.

22.2 Each stage requires separate reasoning. Conflation is a recurring source of error and a fertile ground of appeal.

23 Burden and standard of proof

23.1 The NMC bears the burden of proving the factual allegations relied upon.[72] Fitness to practise proceedings apply the civil standard of proof; the balance of probabilities. That standard applies at the fact-finding stage only. It does not apply to misconduct, impairment or sanction, which involve the exercise of the panel's professional judgement.[73]

23.2 The civil standard applies notwithstanding the seriousness of the allegations or the gravity of the potential consequences.

> Although there is a single civil standard of proof on the balance of probabilities, it is flexible in its application. In particular, the more serious the allegation or the more serious the consequences if the allegation is proved, the stronger must be the evidence before a court will find the allegation proved on the balance of probabilities. Thus the flexibility of the standard lies not in any adjustment to the degree of probability required for an allegation to be proved (such that a more serious allegation has to be proved to a higher degree of probability), but in the strength or quality of the evidence that will in practice be required for an allegation to be proved on the balance of probabilities.[74]

23.3 Practitioners should be careful about taking submissions on the standard too far. Where an act is inherently improbable, a Panel may have to look more critically or anxiously at the evidence,

---

72 FTP rule 30

73 See: *Council for the Regulation of Health Care Professionals v General Medical Council & Biswas* [2006] EWHC 464 (Admin), at [42]ff

74 *AN, R(On the Application of) v Mental Health Review Tribunal (Northern Region)* [2005] EWCA Civ 1605, at [62]

but the standard itself remains "finite and unvarying."[75] As Lord Hoffmann set out in *In re B*:[76]

> There is only one rule of law, namely that the occurrence of the fact in issue must be proved to have been more probable than not. Common sense, not law, requires that in deciding this question, regard should be had, to whatever extent appropriate, to inherent probabilities.

23.4 Once the facts are found proved, the burden does not "shift" in any formal sense, but the practical position changes. At the impairment stage, the tribunal is required to make an evaluative judgement as to current fitness to practise. In doing so, it may properly take account of the presence or absence of evidence from the registrant on matters such as remediation, insight, and current risk. A registrant is not required to prove fitness, but where allegations of a serious or attitudinal nature have been proved, the absence of evidence addressing remediation or insight will weigh heavily against the registrant in the tribunal's assessment.

23.5 This feature is critical for practitioners approaching fitness to practise proceedings from a criminal background to understand. There is no presumption analogous to the presumption of innocence at the impairment stage. Nor is silence or non-engagement a neutral act once adverse findings have been made. The tribunal's task necessarily involves an evaluation of what has, or has not, been put before it by way of evidence addressing *current* fitness to practise.

[75] *In re CD* [2008] UKHL 33. per Lord Carswell at [28]

[76] [2008] UKHL 35, at [15]

24 Statutory grounds

24.1 The NMC's authority to investigate and prosecute arises only where one or more statutory grounds under Article 22 are engaged. The structure of Article 22 matters. The grounds are not loose labels. They are the categories through which Parliament has defined the regulator's enforcement jurisdiction; each ground has a distinct conceptual focus.

25 Misconduct

25.1 Misconduct is the most frequently pleaded statutory ground in fitness to practise proceedings. It is not a catch-all for behaviour that attracts criticism, nor is it synonymous with negligence, error, or poor judgement.

25.2 The seminal definition of misconduct is that of Lord Clyde in *Roylance v General Medical Council*:[77]

> Misconduct is a word of general effect involving some act or omission which falls short of what would be proper in the circumstances. The standard of propriety may often be found by reference to the rules and standards ordinarily required to be followed by a practitioner in the particular circumstances.

25.3 Two features of that definition are central. First, misconduct concerns a falling short of what is "proper"; not merely a failure to achieve optimal or ideal practice. Secondly, the assessment is rooted in "the particular circumstances" faced by the registrant in question at the material time. Misconduct is not assessed in the abstract. It is assessed contextually.

---

77 [1999] UKPC 16, at [38]

25.4 The contextual requirement has real practical force. Panels must identify the specific NMC standards or local rules or procedures said to apply at the material time and must assess the registrant's conduct against those standards as they operated in reality. Evidence of what was required of the registrant in the particular circumstances is therefore imperative. Emergency conditions, systemic pressures, resource constraints, unclear or evolving guidance, and atypical working environments may all play into the assessment and should be addressed in evidence and submissions. An assessment of misconduct that fails to engage with the circumstances in which professionals were operating risks impermissible hindsight reasoning.

25.5 In order to inform the panel's assessment of what would have been proper in the circumstances, the NMC will often adduce in evidence employer policies, procedures or guidance as evidence of the standards said to have governed the registrant's conduct at the material time. In practice, and with striking regularity, those documents post-date the events in question. This is a predictable consequence of the length of time many cases take to reach a final hearing, during which policies are revised, guidance updated, and standards re-articulated or consolidated, with the NMC's evidence-gathering process taking place years after the index events. The approach is improper. Documents created after the alleged conduct are irrelevant to the assessment of misconduct, because FTP proceedings are concerned with whether the registrant's conduct fell seriously below the standards applicable at the time. Practitioners must therefore scrutinise carefully the provenance and dates of any policy evidence relied upon, and be prepared to challenge relevance (i.e. admissibility) where policies relied upon were not in force at the relevant time. Panels should be invited to identify with precision the rules, guidance or professional expectations against which conduct is to be judged.

25.6 Even where established, not every falling short of applicable standards will amount to misconduct. A falling short must "be linked to the practice of medicine or conduct that otherwise brings the profession into disrepute, and it must be serious."[78]

25.7 What is serious? "The adjective 'serious' must be given its proper weight, and in other contexts there has been reference to conduct which would be regarded as deplorable by fellow practitioners. It is of course possible for negligent conduct to amount to serious professional misconduct, but the negligence must be to a high degree." [79]

25.8 The *Nandi* formulation reinforces two propositions.

25.8.1 First, seriousness is not a rhetorical flourish but a substantive threshold. Misconduct commonly arises where conduct reflects attitudinal or ethical failings. Dishonesty, abuse of professional position, exploitation of vulnerability, serious boundary violations, discriminatory conduct, harassment, safeguarding failures, and serious breaches of confidentiality are paradigm examples. In such cases, seriousness lies not only in the patient-facing outcome, but in what the conduct reveals about integrity, trustworthiness, and adherence to core professional values.

25.8.2 Second, while negligence and misconduct may overlap, they are not interchangeable categorisations. Ordinary negligence does not, without more, amount to misconduct.

---

[78] *Meadow v General Medical Council* [2006] EWCA Civ 1390, at [200]

[79] *Nandi v General Medical Council* [2004] EWHC 2317 (Admin), at [31]

25.9 It is well settled that misconduct can arise from "omission or commission".[80] In *R (on the application of Calhaem) v General Medical Council*,[81] Jackson J distilled two principles from the authorities:

> (1) Mere negligence does not constitute 'misconduct' [...] Nevertheless, and depending upon the circumstances, negligent acts or omissions which are particularly serious may amount to 'misconduct'.
>
> (2) A single negligent act or omission is less likely to cross the threshold of 'misconduct' than multiple acts or omissions. Nevertheless, and depending upon the circumstances, a single negligent act or omission, if particularly grave, could be characterised as 'misconduct'.

25.10 Misconduct is therefore neither dependent upon multiplicity, nor excluded by singularity. The question is one of gravity, assessed contextually. A pattern of negligent acts may cumulatively cross the threshold. Equally, a single act may do so if it is sufficiently serious in its nature or consequences: "serious professional misconduct for this purpose may take the form, not only of acts of bad faith or other moral turpitude, but also of incompetence or negligence of a high degree."[82]

25.11 The same approach was endorsed in *R (on the application of Vali) v General Optical Council*,[83] where Ouseley J stated that "mere negligence does not of itself show that the act was misconduct. A higher degree of gravity than mere carelessness

---

80 *Doughty v General Dental Council* [1988] AC 164, at 173

81 [2007] EWHC 2606 (Admin), at [39]

82 *Meadow* at [201]

83 [2011] EWHC 310 (Admin), at [28]

is required. I also note and agree that a single act is less likely to cross the threshold of misconduct but that depends of course on the gravity of the act."

25.12 There remain divergent views on whether misconduct properly encompasses any moral element, with legal advice to panels occasionally suggesting that there is. In *Spencer v General Osteopathic Council*,[84] Irwin J said that misconduct does carry "an implication of moral blameworthiness, and a degree of opprobrium is likely to be conveyed to the ordinary intelligent citizen". In *Meadow*, Auld LJ echoed the observation that "in other contexts it has been referred to as "conduct which would be regarded as deplorable by fellow practitioners"."[85]

25.13 In fact, moral blameworthiness is not a necessary ingredient: morally inapposite behaviour may amount to misconduct; not all misconduct will be morally inapposite. In *Remedy UK*,[86] the principles from the authorities were summarised thus:

> Misconduct is of two principal kinds. First, it may involve sufficiently serious misconduct in the exercise of professional practice such that it can properly be described as misconduct going to fitness to practise. Second, it can involve conduct of a morally culpable or otherwise disgraceful kind which may, and often will, occur outwith the course of professional practice itself, but which brings disgrace upon the doctor and thereby prejudices the reputation of the profession.

---

84 [2012] EWHC 3147 (Admin), at [23]

85 *Meadow* at [200]

86 *Remedy UK Ltd, R (On the Application of) v General Medical Council* [2010] EWHC 1245 (Admin), at [37]

> [...]
>
> Conduct falls into the second limb if it is dishonourable or disgraceful or attracts some kind of opprobrium; that fact may be sufficient to bring the profession of medicine into disrepute. It matters not whether such conduct is directly related to the exercise of professional skills.

25.14 The import of moral judgement is invariably unhelpful. "It is settled that serious professional misconduct does not require moral turpitude. Gross professional negligence can fall within it. Something more is required than a degree of negligence enough to give rise to civil liability but not calling for the opprobrium that inevitably attaches to the disciplinary offence."[87] Misconduct "is not restricted to conduct which is morally blameworthy"[88] and ""moral blameworthiness" plays no part in the definition."[89]

25.15 In delivering their decisions on misconduct, panels must articulate the standards relied upon, explain how the conduct fell seriously below those standards, and justify why the seriousness threshold is met in the circumstances of the case. Formulaic recitation that "this conduct fell seriously below the standard expected" is insufficient; properly reasoned findings of misconduct are essential to form a logical foundation upon which to evaluate impairment and sanction.

26 Lack of competence

26.1 Lack of competence is "conceptually separate both from negligence and from misconduct. It connotes a standard of

[87] *Preiss v General Dental Council* [2001] 1WLR 1926

[88] *Nandi*, at [32]

[89] *Benn v General Medical Council* [2025] EWHC 87 (Admin), at [79]

professional performance which is unacceptably low and which (save in exceptional circumstances) has been demonstrated by reference to a fair sample of the doctor's work."[90] Lack of competence is concerned with professional knowledge and skills.

26.2 The assessment is objective and contextual. In *Holton v General Medical Council*,[91] the court explained that the appropriate benchmark is the standard applicable to the post to which the practitioner was appointed and the work they were carrying out. The test is the standard to be expected of a competent practitioner in the circumstances.

26.3 The assessment is deliberately impersonal. It is irrelevant that the practitioner has not had sufficient training; professional performance is no less deficient because the practitioner has not been sufficiently trained or educated.[92] Facts personal to the practitioner, including education, training and personality, are irrelevant to the threshold question of deficiency. Those matters may become relevant later.

26.4 At the same time, competence is assessed contextually. External factors such as pressure of work, lack of resources, and professional isolation due to absence of colleagues are relevant. Performance is assessed against what can reasonably be expected in the circumstances.[93] By contrast, professional isolation attributable to the practitioner's own personality or behaviour is not a relevant mitigating factor.

---

90 *Calhaem,* at [39]

91 [2006] EWHC 2960 (Admin), at [70] – [71]

92 *Holton*, at [74]

93 *Holton*, at [75]

26.5 As with misconduct, a single instance of negligent treatment, unless very serious indeed, will rarely suffice. "No single instance of negligence or unacceptable care would be sufficient to found a conclusion of "professional incompetence". Hence for both purposes, a breach of the Code of Practice is a starting point and is relevant, but cannot be definitive or indeed even raise a presumption that "professional incompetence" or "unacceptable professional conduct" is made out."[94]

26.6 In practice, lack of competence is often pleaded in the alternative to misconduct. That custom carries dangers. The higher courts have warned against stretching lack of competence to capture conduct which is more properly characterised as misconduct. Lack of competence "should not be contorted so that it is a mere synonym for "misconduct" in practice. [It] is more in contrast to than coterminous with misconduct. It is intended at least to be different in that one would often, if not normally, expect to find a pattern of conduct underlying the allegation of deficient professional performance."[95]

26.7 Although the same facts may sometimes justify charges under both heads, care is required. Simply re-labelling misconduct as lack of competence risks doctrinal confusion and unfairness.

27 Health

27.1 Allegations of impairment by reason of health are concerned not with professional standards or culpability, but with whether a registrant's physical or mental health condition currently impairs their ability to practise safely and effectively. The question in such cases is whether the registrant's health

---

[94] *Spencer*, at [24]

[95] *Vali*, at [28]

condition gives rise to a present or future risk to patients, the public, or the registrant themselves. Fault, blame, or moral judgement play no part in the analysis.

27.2 Proceedings relating to impairment by reason of health must be conducted in private,[96] unless (exceptionally) a panel is satisfied that the need to protect the privacy of the registrant is outweighed by the public interest.[97] Article 8 interests are firmly engaged by medical evidence and there is limited public value in exposing confidential health information. The presumption of privacy does not, however, alter the panel's obligation to give proper reasons.

27.3 The assessment of impairment in health cases is clinical and evidential. Panels must identify a relevant health condition, supported by cogent medical evidence, and must then determine whether that condition currently impairs fitness to practise. A diagnosis alone is insufficient. The critical question is functional impact: how the condition affects the registrant's ability to practise safely and reliably.

27.4 Insight, compliance with treatment, engagement with occupational health, and prognosis are evidentially significant. A registrant may have a serious health condition and yet not be impaired if it is well-managed and does not pose a risk. Conversely, impairment may be established where a condition is untreated, unstable, or poorly managed, even if no harm has yet occurred.

27.5 Sanctions in health cases are protective and supportive. Conditions of practice are commonly appropriate where risk can be managed. Suspension may be justified where there is no

96 FTP rule 19(2)

97 FTP rule 19(2A)

safe alternative. A striking-off order cannot be imposed where fitness to practise is impaired due to health, unless the registrant has been subject to a substantive suspension or a conditions of practice order for a continuous period of two years.[98]

28 Language impairment

28.1 Concerns about a registrant's knowledge of English engage fitness to practise where they raise issues of patient safety, professional effectiveness, or the ability to practise safely in the UK healthcare system.

28.2 Where language competence is in issue, the regulator may direct the registrant to undertake a language assessment. The purpose of such a direction is evidential. The outcome of the assessment is ordinarily treated as the primary objective evidence of language competence.

28.3 Directions must be given in writing and will specify the form of assessment, the timeframe, and the period for providing results. The regulator ordinarily meets the cost of the assessment it directs. In practice, IELTS is commonly specified, though OET results are accepted where obtained independently.

28.4 Failure to comply with a direction has evidential consequences. FTP rule 31(6A) permits a panel to draw such inference as it considers appropriate from non-compliance. Non-compliance does not amount to automatic proof of impairment, but it may support adverse inference where the failure is unexplained or unjustified.

[98] Article 29(6)

29 Conviction and caution cases

29.1 Where a registrant has received a criminal conviction or caution, the fact of that outcome provides an established factual foundation for regulatory proceedings. The tribunal's function is to determine whether, in light of the conviction or caution, the registrant's fitness to practise is currently impaired and, if so, what response is required to meet the statutory objectives.

29.2 A certificate of conviction stands as conclusive proof of a conviction,[99] unless the registrant can demonstrate that they are not the person named in the certificate.[100]

29.3 Where a registrant is absolutely or conditionally discharged by the criminal court upon conviction, the NMC cannot proceed on a conviction basis; the "conviction of that offence is to be deemed not to be a conviction for any purpose other than the purposes of [...] the proceedings in which the order is made."[101]

29.4 FTP rule 31(2)(b), which stems from power conferred under Article 32(2)(p) of the 2001 Order, reflects the well-established principle that where statute provides for professional consequences to follow a conviction, the effect of the statute "is to preclude the practitioner from denying the truth of any facts necessarily implied in the conviction."[102]

---

[99] FTP rule 31(2)(a)

[100] FTP rule 31(3)

[101] s.82(2) *Sentencing Act 2020*

[102] *Kirk v Royal College of Veterinary Surgeons* [2004] UKPC 4, at [6]

29.5 In *Wray v General Osteopathic Council*,[103] the High Court summarised the position thus:

> The authorities have consistently held that where statutory provision is made for disciplinary bodies to attach professional consequences to a criminal conviction, the effect of the statute has been to preclude the practitioner from denying the truth of any facts necessarily implied in the conviction [...] That includes cases where conviction is based on a guilty plea [..] What the practitioner cannot do is to relitigate the conviction as to the facts.
>
> It is both unnecessary and undesirable to re-try a criminal case – unnecessary where the facts have already been pleaded and established to the criminal standard, and undesirable because of the public interest in the finality of criminal procedure. The only issue left for a disciplinary body is the relevance of conviction and sentence to the professional standard of the participant.

29.6 The irrefutable factual basis of a conviction is not limited to the bare particulars contained in the certificate of conviction, but extends to the factual matrix as articulated in the sentencing remarks of the sentencing judge. Allowing a registrant to dispute those facts would undermine the integrity of the regulatory system.[104] Within the NMC scheme, therefore, evidence contradicting the verdict, or seeking to re-litigate the criminal trial, is inadmissible.

---

[103] [2020] EWHC 3409 (QB), at [32] – [33]

[104] *Achina v General Pharmaceutical Council* [2021] EWHC 415 (Admin), at [84]

29.7 That does not mean that all ancillary material is treated as conclusive, nor that evidence beyond the certificate of conviction or caution is of no value. "Both the [regulator] and the practitioner may adduce evidence about the underlying facts upon which the conviction is based, provided that the facts which such evidence is relevant to prove are not inconsistent with the finding that the respondent was guilty of the offence."[105]

29.8 In practice, the regulator will often seek to rely not only on a certificate of conviction but also on material arising from criminal proceedings such as an MG5 case summary. Practitioners should be alert to the distinction. An MG5 is not admissible evidence in a criminal trial and is not a judicial finding of fact within the meaning of FTP rule 31(2)(b). Although the broader admissibility rules in fitness to practise proceedings will often permit its admission, it does not have the same evidential status as a certificate of conviction or sentencing remarks. It may assist with context, but it cannot displace or expand the facts necessarily implied by the conviction itself.

29.9 The existence of a conviction or caution does not answer the impairment question. That assessment remains evaluative and forward-looking. The tribunal must consider seriousness, relevance to professional practice, insight, remediation, risk of repetition, and public confidence.

29.10 Not all convictions carry the same regulatory weight. The role of the NMC "in protecting patients involves different considerations from those taken into account by the criminal courts when passing sentence. For example, an offence of dishonesty or of indecency committed by a [medical professional] will have implications in the context of medical

---

[105] *Kirk,* at [8]

practice that go well beyond the considerations that the courts will take into account. What may appear relatively trivial in the context of the general criminal law may be quite serious in the context of medical practice."[106] Offences involving dishonesty, violence, sexual misconduct, abuse, or safeguarding will ordinarily engage impairment, but careful reasoning is required in every case.

29.11 Cautions require particular care. Although not convictions, cautions involve an admission of offending and are expressly recognised within the statutory scheme. Their regulatory significance depends on context and consequence.

29.12 The boundary is clear. Registrants may advance mitigation and contextual explanation relevant to impairment and sanction, but they may not deny or undermine the factual basis of a conviction or caution. To do so is impermissible, inconsistent with settled authority, and liable to be curtailed.

29.13 A registrant who is subject to a sentence imposed by a criminal court is likely to be found impaired: "as a general principle, where a practitioner has been convicted of a serious criminal offence or offences he should not be permitted to resume his practice until he has satisfactorily completed his sentence."[107] That principle, however, "cannot be applied as if it were a

[106] Dame Janet Smith, *Fifth Shipman Report,* at [23.34]

[107] *CHRE v General Dental Council and Fleischmann* [2005] EWHC 87 (Admin), at [54]

rule"[108] and may in any event "bow to the particular circumstances of a particular case."[109]

30 Determinations by other bodies

30.1 Article 22 permits regulatory intervention where there has been an adverse determination by another professional or regulatory body, whether in the UK or overseas. The rationale is protective rather than punitive. Where a registrant has been found impaired by another relevant regulator, the question for the NMC is whether that determination has implications for the registrant's nursing or midwifery practice in the UK, or nursing associate practice in England, such that the register no longer accurately reflects public safety, trustworthiness, or professional standards.

30.2 In such cases, the NMC does not proceed on the basis of automatic transposition. Decision-makers must consider the scope and nature of the other regulator's determination, the factual background to it, and how closely the issues relate to nursing or midwifery practice within the NMC's statutory remit. This involves an evaluative assessment of the underlying facts, any relevant contextual features, and whether those matters were considered by the other body. The central questions remain whether the registrant presents a current risk of harm to the public, whether the determination engages public confidence in the nursing or midwifery professions, and whether regulatory action is required to maintain proper professional standards.

---

108 *Professional Standards Authority v General Dental Council & Patel* [2024] EWHC 243 (Admin), at [19]

109 *Opare v Nursing and Midwifery Council* [2019] EWHC 1851 (Admin), at [30]

30.3 Procedurally, these cases require particular care. Determinations of other regulators are capable of being admitted in evidence, but they do not displace the tribunal's obligation to exercise independent judgement. FTP rule 31(4) provides that a signed certificate of another body's determination is admissible "as prima facie evidence of the facts referred to" in that determination. That evidential status is significant, but by no means determinative of impairment. The tribunal must still decide what weight to attach to the material, bearing in mind differences in regulatory frameworks, standards, purposes, and professional context.

31 Impairment

31.1 Impairment is the central battleground in many FTP proceedings. It is the point at which past misdoings ossify into present regulatory consequence.

31.2 The assessment of impairment is a separate exercise to the consideration of misconduct, and does not follow automatically: "not [...] every case of misconduct found at stage 1 must automatically mean that the practitioner's fitness to practice is impaired. [...] There must always be situations in which a Panel can properly conclude that the act of misconduct was an isolated error on the part of a medical practitioner and that the chance of it being repeated in the future is so remote that his or her fitness to practice has not been impaired." [110]

31.3 Crucially, the assessment of impairment is conducted in the present tense irrespective of the age of the concerns found proved or admitted. The question to be asked and answered by

[110] *Cohen v General Medical Council* [2008] EWHC 581 Admin, at [63] – [64] [sic]

the Panel: is the registrant's fitness to practise *currently* impaired?

31.4 As Sir Anthony Clarke said, in *Meadow v General Medical Council*:[111]

> "In short, the purpose of FTP proceedings is not to punish the practitioner for past misdoings but to protect the public against the acts and omissions of those who are not fit to practise. The FTPP thus looks forward not back. However, in order to form a view as to the fitness of a person to practise today, it is evident that it will have to take account of the way in which the person concerned has acted or failed to act in the past."

31.5 NMC guidance and the jurisprudence commonly distinguishes two 'components' of impairment i.e. two gateways through which impairment may be established.

<u>The Personal Component</u>

31.6 The personal component concerns current risk to patients and the risk of repetition. It is commonly analysed through the *Cohen* questions: whether the concern is readily remediable; whether it has been remedied; and whether it is highly unlikely to be repeated.

31.7 These are the key questions to be addressed in evidence and submissions. Evidence of training, supervision, reflective work, changed practice and testimonials may all be relevant, but panels scrutinise such material closely. Generic courses and formulaic reflections carry limited weight unless they

[111] [2006] EWCA Civ 1390, at [3]

demonstrate genuine learning connected to the specific failings found proved.

Insight

31.7.1 Insight is frequently decisive. Insight is not simply regret. It requires acceptance of what went wrong, a demonstrable understanding on the part of the registrant of why it went wrong, and an informed understanding of the impact on others, and what could be done to prevent recurrence.

31.7.2 Continued denial or minimisation in the face of factual findings commonly undermines arguments that personal impairment has resolved. A perennial difficulty in defending FTP proceedings occurs where a registrant has denied that conduct took place, but hours or days later is subject to adverse factual findings and required to address the panel on insight into conduct which may still be denied.

31.7.3 Registrants are not required to evidence a volte face of position; insight is not dependent upon accepting the panel's stage 1 findings:

> I think that it is too much to expect of an accused member of a profession who has doughtily defended an allegation on the ground that he did not do it suddenly to undergo a Damascene conversion in the impairment phase following a factual finding that he did do it.
>
> It is for this reason that explicit admissions of culpability tend not to be given in the impairment and sanctions phase. Rather, language alters to the passive voice and statements

> in the genre of "I am sorry if what I have said has caused you to take offence" are made.
>
> That is some distance away from admitting explicitly the truth of what the tribunal had found proved. In my judgment, in the absence of any significant hiatus between the factual finding and the impairment/sanctions phase in which full reflection can be undergone, that is as much as can reasonably be expected of an accused professional who has defended the case on the ground that he did not do what was alleged.[112]

31.7.4 In *Sayer v General Osteopathic Council*,[113] Morris J distilled the relevant authorities to these propositions:

> (1) Insight is concerned with future risk of repetition. To this extent, it is to be distinguished from remorse for the past conduct.
>
> (2) Denial of misconduct is not a reason to increase sanction: *Awan* §38.
>
> (3) It is wrong to equate maintenance of innocence with lack of insight. Denial of misconduct is not an absolute bar to a finding of insight. Admitting misconduct is not a condition precedent to establishing that the registrant understands the gravity of the offending and is unlikely to repeat it: *Motala* §34 and *Awan* §38.

---

112 *General Medical Council v Awan* [2020] EWHC 1553 (Admin), at [37] – [40]

113 [2021] EWHC 370 (Admin), at [25]

(4) However attitude to the underlying allegation is properly to be taken into account when weighing up insight: *Motala* §34 Where the registrant continues to deny impropriety, that makes it more difficult for him to demonstrate insight. The underlying importance of insight and its relationship with denial of misconduct was usefully analysed by Andrew Baker J in *Khetyar* (at §49) as follows:

> "Of course, no sanction was to be imposed on him for his denials as such; however, insight requires that motivations and triggers be identified and understood, and if that is possible at all without there first being an acceptance that what happened did happen it will be very rare, and any assessment of ongoing risk must play close attention to the doctor's current understanding of and attitude towards what he has done.".

(5) The assessment of the extent of insight is a matter for the tribunal, weighing all the evidence and having heard the registrant. The Court should be slow to interfere: *Motala* §§30 and 31.

31.7.5 Although oral evidence is not an absolute requirement, absence from the hearing or silence commonly makes it harder to demonstrate insight, and risks the absence of insight being later identified as an aggravating feature in the consideration of sanction:

In circumstances where the Appellant did not admit the misconduct and had not apologised, it

> would have been open to the Tribunal to infer that there was a lack of remorse and/or insight and to treat that as an additional aggravating factor. [...] In those circumstances, where there was no evidence of insight or remorse, the weight to be attached to the lack of likelihood of repetition is likely to be substantially diminished.[114]

31.7.6 Insight is ultimately a matter of evaluative judgement for the tribunal based on all the evidence. In the absence of a registrant, a panel will not "necessarily be disabled from making the findings it needs to make on insight, or bound to find that the registrant lacks it."[115] Written material and third-party evidence may all contribute. There will, however, be cases where the registrant's own oral evidence is the best, or only, convincing evidence available.

31.7.7 In *Henderson v General Teaching Council for England*,[116] the court rejected the proposition that an absent registrant who admits misconduct and apologises through counsel necessarily demonstrates insight. Late or pressured admissions, without explanation or engagement, are not equivalent to early, unprompted acceptance.

---

114 *Sidhu v Bar Standards Board* [2026] EWHC 25 (Admin), at [82]

115 *Professional Standards Authority v Health and Care Professional Council & Doree* [2017] EWCA Civ 319, at [38]

116 [2012] EWHC 1505 (Admin)

Remediation

31.7.8 In practice, there is a persuasive burden on the registrant to demonstrate that steps have been taken to strengthen or remedy deficiencies. In *Kimmance v General Medical Council*,[117] Kerr J put the reality thus:

> There was indeed no evidence of insight and remediation in this case. I do not much like those jargon words. They do not do much to illuminate the reality, which is that a doctor or other professional who has done wrong has to look at his or her conduct with a self-critical eye, acknowledge fault, say sorry and convince a panel that there is real reason to believe he or she has learned a lesson from the experience. Nine times out of ten, you cannot do that if you do not turn up to the hearing. The panel will want to ask questions.

31.7.9 While, again, the registrant is not required to abandon previous denials at the impairment stage, "it is very difficult to remediate, and to show that what motivated and triggered the misconduct has been identified and understood, without an acceptance that what happened did happen."[118]

31.7.10 The NMC publishes guidance on impairment and strengthened practice, to which deference is paid. Remediation is not about box-ticking. Panels will look for evidence that the registrant has changed how

[117] [2016] EWHC 1808, at [66]

[118] *Safdar v General Medical Council* [2025] EWHC 3176 (Admin), at [51]

they practise, how they think, or how they respond to risk. Where remediation is asserted but not evidenced, or where it is superficial, arguments that personal impairment has resolved are unlikely to succeed.

31.7.11 From a practical perspective, remediation needs to be approached deliberately and early, with an eye to evidencing real change. Practitioners should identify precisely what the panel is likely to find went wrong, isolate the underlying causes, and then take concrete steps to address them. That will often include targeted training directly linked to the failing, changes to working practices, supervision or mentoring arrangements, and reflective work that grapples candidly with impact and learning rather than rehearsing platitudes. Certificates of training alone are rarely sufficient without an explanation of what was learned and how it has altered practice; reflective pieces should engage with the findings rather than skirt around them; testimonials are most persuasive where they come from supervisors who understand the concerns and can speak to observed change over time.

31.7.12 Above all, panels look for coherence between what is said and what has been done. Remediation that appears reactive, generic or assembled shortly before a hearing will usually be afforded limited weight. Sustained steps taken well in advance, capable of being and in fact tested through questioning, are far more likely to demonstrate reduced risk and unimpaired fitness to practise.

31.7.13 Often, the most cogent evidence of remediation is the absence of repetition since the index events. Given that proceedings invariably take several years to reach final hearing, those registrants who are able to practise pending final hearing are well-placed to demonstrate in practice that they have learnt their lesson.

Remorse

31.7.14 Remorse may be relevant, but expressions of regret carry little weight if they are unaccompanied by insight or remediation, particularly where they follow sustained denial. Panels will look beyond words to substance: what has been learned, what has changed, and why repetition is now unlikely.

The Public Component

31.8 The public component concerns confidence in the profession and in the regulatory system. Frequently, registrants are considered impaired on this ground alone; where personal risk is low but a declaration of impairment is nevertheless required to uphold professional standards.

> Where a FTPP considers that fitness to practise is impaired for such reasons, and that a firm declaration of professional standards so as to promote public confidence in that medical practitioner and the profession generally is required, the efforts made by the practitioner to address his problems and to reduce the risk of recurrence of such misconduct in the future may be of far less significance than in other cases.[119]

[119] *Yeong v General Medical Council* [2009] EWHC 1923 (Admin), at [51]

31.9 The modern approach is anchored in the Fifth Shipman Report as endorsed in *CHRE v NMC and Grant*:[120] the panel asks whether the proved matters show that the registrant has in the past acted, and/or is liable in the future to act, so as to (a) put patients at unwarranted risk of harm, (b) bring the profession into disrepute, (c) breach a fundamental tenet of the profession, and/or (d) act dishonestly. Consistently with *Grant*, the panel must consider not only current risk but also whether the need to uphold proper professional standards and maintain public confidence would be undermined if impairment were not found in the particular circumstances.

31.10 Public confidence is not, however, a licence for moral condemnation. Panels must explain why, in the particular case, the absence of a finding would undermine trust or standards. Conclusory invocations are insufficient.

31.11 Panels should be reminded that a finding of misconduct alone can be sufficient to demonstrate that the NMC has acted appropriately and to discharge the public interest. A finding of impairment is not always required. In *Uppal*,[121] the Court took the view that the FTP process and a finding of misconduct was itself sufficient to provide sufficient protection:

> Professional standards have upheld, and public confidence in the profession maintained, by the fact that Dr Uppal has undergone a rigorous disciplinary assessment of her fitness to practise, resulting in a finding of misconduct on her record.

---

[120] [2011] EWHC 927 (Admin)

[121] *Professional Standards Authority v General Medical Council & Uppal* [2015] EWHC 1304 (Admin), at [34]

31.12 Certain categories of misconduct have been the subject of particular commentary by the higher courts on the question of impairment and are, in all but exceptional cases, likely to necessitate a finding of impairment on public interest grounds.

Dishonesty

31.13 Though the courts have made clear that "not every act of dishonesty results in impairment,"[122] it is trite that "for all professional men and women, a finding of dishonesty lies at the top end of the spectrum of gravity of misconduct [...] In cases of proven dishonesty, the balance can be expected to fall down on the side of maintaining public confidence in the profession."[123]

31.14 In *General Medical Council v Armstrong*,[124] Lane J echoed the sentiment:

> the consequences of a finding of dishonesty in the professional regulatory context are likely to be so profound, in terms of the overarching regulatory objective, that the factors on the other side, viewed as a whole, will need to be extremely strong, in order for a finding of no impairment to be justified. Competing factors of the required overall strength are unlikely to be frequently encountered.

31.15 In practice, "it will therefore be an unusual case where dishonesty is not found to impair fitness to practise."[125]

---

[122] *Uppal*, at [27]

[123] *Khan v General Medical Council* [2015] EWHC 301 (Admin), at [6] – [8]

[124] [2021] EWHC 1658 (Admin), at [53]

[125] *Professional Standards Authority v Health and Care Professions Council & Ghaffar* [2014] EWHC 2723 (Admin), at [46]

Dishonesty, however, encompasses a broad range of behaviours: "some criminal, some not; some destroying trust instantly, others merely undermining it to a greater or lesser extent."[126] Panels must engage with the nature of the dishonesty when consider the extent to which the public interest is engaged.

<u>Sexual misconduct</u>

31.16 Sexual misconduct is similarly treated as falling at the top end of seriousness. Such conduct "undermines public trust in the profession. It is accordingly more difficult to remediate than poor clinical performance and mitigation is afforded limited weight as the reputation of the profession is more important than the fortunes of the individual member."[127]

31.17 As with dishonesty, however, "there must be an assessment of where an act of sexual misconduct, albeit inherently serious, falls on the scale of gravity."[128]

32 Sanction

32.1 If impairment is found, the tribunal must determine what, if any, sanction is necessary to meet the statutory objectives; to protect the public, to maintain confidence in the profession and in the regulatory regime, and to uphold proper professional standards.

32.2 As Sir Anthony Clarke MR explained in *Meadow*, fitness to practise proceedings exist "not to punish the practitioner for past misdoings but to protect the public against the acts and

---

[126] *Lusinga v Nursing And Midwifery Council* [2017] EWHC 1458 (Admin), at [103]

[127] *Sadiq v General Medical Council* [2025] EWHC 3062 (Admin), at [87]

[128] *Sidhu v Bar Standards Board* [2026] EWHC 25 (Admin), at [38]

omissions of those who are not fit to practise".[129] Practitioners are wise to remember that "the question of sanction for a regulator is not the same as that of a court imposing retributive punishment."[130] Comparisons with criminal sentencing are of limited utility and must be approached with caution.

32.3 The guiding principle for sanction is proportionality. Any order imposed must go no further than is necessary to meet the statutory aims. This is reflected both in the case law and in the structure of the NMC's Sanctions Guidance. Panels are required to consider sanctions in ascending order of severity, starting with the least restrictive outcome and moving upwards only if a lesser sanction would be insufficient to protect the public or the wider public interest.

32.4 In *Giele v General Medical Council,*[131] the court emphasised that the public interest consideration at the sanction stage is not a factor which uniformly weighs against the interests of a registrant; "the existence of a public interest in not ending the career of a competent doctor will play a part" and that, where erasure is not inevitable, "the skills of the practitioner are a relevant factor" in determining the proportionate regulatory outcome.

Sanctions Guidance

32.5 The NMC's indicative sanctions guidance[132] is an important and routinely relied upon tool in sanction decision-making. It promotes consistency and transparency, but it does not displace

---

[129] *Meadow*, at [32]

[130] *Mubarak v General Medical Council* [2008] EWHC 2830 (Admin), at [8]

[131] [2005] EWHC 2143 (Admin)

[132] SAN-1 to SAN-6

the panel's independent judgement. The courts have repeatedly emphasised its status as guidance rather than a binding tariff.

32.6 In *Bawa-Garba v General Medical Council*,[133] the Lord Chief Justice explained that the Sanctions Guidance contains "very useful guidance to help provide consistency in approach and outcome" and "should always be consulted", but that it is "no more than that, non-statutory guidance, the relevance and application of which will always depend on the precise circumstances of the particular case". The same point was made in *Atkinson v General Medical Council*,[134] where the court remarked that Indicative Sanctions Guidance "is just that: guidance". Panels must take it into account, and departures may require explanation, but it is not the source of legal obligation.

32.7 Where a panel does opt to depart from the "authoritative steer"[135] of sanctions guidance, it must give clear reasons for doing so.[136]

32.8 In practice, the sanctions guidance provides the framework within which panels reason their way through sanction. It identifies aggravating and mitigating factors, explains the purpose and typical use of different orders, and assists panels in articulating why a particular outcome is necessary and proportionate in the individual case.

---

[133] [2018] EWCA Civ 1879, at [83]

[134] [2009] EWHC 3636 (Admin)

[135] *General Medical Council v Khetyar* [2018] EWHC 813 (Admin), at [22]

[136] *Professional Standards Authority v Health and Care Professional Council & Doree* [2017] EWCA Civ 319, at [29]

Available sanctions

32.9 Taking no further action is available but is exceptional in practice. It is reserved for cases where impairment is found but the panel concludes that the statutory objectives are nevertheless met without any order, typically because the risk is addressed and the public interest does not require further marking.

32.10 It is open to a panel to "undertake mediation of the matter."[137] Though available as a matter of law, and having been amended from "refer the matter to Screeners for mediation or itself undertake mediation"[138] with effect from 28 January 2019, this remedy does not feature in the NMC's sanctions guidance.

32.11 A caution order may be imposed for a period of between one and five years.[139] It is appropriate where impairment is at the lower end of the spectrum, there is no ongoing risk requiring restriction, but a formal marking of the misconduct is needed to uphold standards and public confidence.

32.12 A conditions of practice order may be imposed for up to three years.[140] It is generally appropriate where the concerns are capable of remediation and can be managed safely through workable, measurable and enforceable conditions, usually in cases involving clinical or performance shortcomings rather than fundamentally attitudinal failings. Practitioners should pay particular care when proposing conditions to ensure that they are targeted at the underlying concerns, workable in practice, and that progress can be meaningfully monitored.

---

[137] Article 29(4)

[138] *Nursing and Midwifery (Amendment) Order*, SI 2018/838, Sch.1 para.21

[139] Article 29(5)(d)

[140] Article 29(5)(c)

Conditions may not be formulated with such stringency as to amount to *de facto* suspension,[141] and must relate exclusively to the mischief in the case.[142]

32.13 A suspension order may be imposed for up to 12 months.[143] It is appropriate where the conduct is serious and requires temporary removal from practice to protect the public or to mark seriousness, but where remediation remains a realistic prospect and the registrant is not regarded as fundamentally incompatible with continued registration.

32.14 A striking-off order is the most severe sanction.[144] It is reserved for the most serious cases where public protection, the maintenance of confidence, or the declaration and upholding of proper standards require permanent removal from the register. A striking-off order cannot be imposed at the substantive FTP hearing where fitness to practise is impaired due to health, lack of competence or insufficient knowledge of English, but may be imposed subsequently where a registrant has been subject to a substantive suspension or a conditions of practice order for a continuous period of two years.[145]

Aggravating and mitigating features

32.15 The panel will look to the guidance and identify any relevant aggravating or mitigating features from the non-exhaustive list therein. The context of the underlying conduct, environmental

141 *Udom v General Medical Council* [2009] EWHC 3242 (Admin), at [31]

142 *Carruthers v General Medical Council* [2003] UKPC 42, at [24] – [26]

143 Article 29(5)(b)

144 Article 29(5)(a)

145 Article 29(6)

pressures and isolated nature of concerns may properly play a part in the panel's reasoning at this stage.

32.16 Practitioners are well-placed to note that "matters of [personal] mitigation are likely to be of considerably less significance in regulatory proceedings than to a court imposing retributive justice, because the overarching concern of the professional regulator is the protection of the public."[146] Matters such as personal hardship, health difficulties, financial consequences, or the impact of sanction on a registrant's career may attract sympathy, but they do not address risk, standards, or confidence. As the higher courts have repeatedly emphasised, the personal impact of sanction is an inevitable consequence of regulation, not a factor capable of outweighing the public interest. Personal mitigation may inform the choice between otherwise appropriate sanctions, or the length or structure of an order, but it cannot displace the need for a sanction that adequately protects the public and maintains professional standards.

32.17 The fact that a registrant has denied the allegations, or maintained innocence, is not an aggravating factor in itself; an accused professional is entitled to advance any defence they wish and to have a fair trial of that defence "without facing the jeopardy, if the defence is disbelieved, of further charges or enhanced sanctions."[147] While a panel may properly take into account the extent of insight demonstrated after findings are made, sanction must not be aggravated simply because the registrant put the regulator to proof.

---

[146] *General Medical Council v Jagjivan & Anor* [2017] EWHC 1247 (Admin), at [40(vii)]

[147] *General Medical Council v Awan* [2020] EWHC 1553 (Admin), at [38]

Sanction submissions

32.18 Sanction submissions should be structured, principled and evidence-led. Practitioners should root submissions on sanction in the applicable provisions of the sanctions guidance, particularly insofar as the guidance addresses specific categories of misconduct. Panels will expect parties to address seriousness (mitigation and aggravation), proportionality, the statutory objectives, and the available range of outcomes. Submissions should explain why lesser sanctions would or would not be sufficient, and why the proposed outcome is necessary to protect the public and the wider public interest.

32.19 The application of sanction principles varies by category of case. While the overarching framework remains constant, panels approach different types of misconduct in distinct ways. Practitioners will be assisted by the category-specific guidance provided by the NMC.

32.20 Certain misconduct is overwhelmingly likely to result in strike-off in all but exceptional cases. Particularly, dishonesty,[148] sexual misconduct[149] and conviction for serious criminal offences.

33 The role of the legal assessor

33.1 Panels are supported by a legal assessor, but responsibility for findings, impairment and sanction rests squarely with the panel. The assessor's function is advisory, not determinative. In *Haikel v General Medical Council*,[150] the Privy Council confirmed that

---

[148] *Photay, R (On the Application of) v General Dental Council* [2023] EWHC 661 (Admin), at [45]

[149] *Sadiq v General Medical Council* [2025] EWHC 3062 (Admin), at [87]

[150] [2002] UKPC 37

while a legal assessor may express a view on the law, the committee remains free to accept it, reject it, or attach such weight to it as it considers appropriate. The 'LA' is not a judge. "He gives legal advice but does not give directions as such and does not sum up the evidence to the Panel."[151]

33.2 In *Libman v General Medical Council*,[152] the Privy Council explained that the assessor advises on the law, but the panel is master of both law and fact. On challenge, the question is not whether the advice resembled a judicial summing-up, but whether it was of sufficient significance to vitiate the decision.

33.3 The courts have also emphasised that the legal assessor's role in providing advice is not confined to posing abstract questions. In *Mahfouz v General Medical Council*,[153] the Court of Appeal made clear that where issues of fairness or natural justice arise, the legal assessor should ordinarily do more than frame questions for the panel. The legal assessor is often better placed than lay members to articulate the correct legal approach, including the perspective of the fair-minded observer, and should give substantive advice on the applicable legal tests, while leaving the ultimate decision to the panel. This line of authority is reflected in the FTP rules; rule 18(6) specifically empowers the legal assessor to "give a preliminary opinion for the purpose of resolving questions of law or admissibility of evidence."

[151] *Gopakumar v General Medical Council* [2008] EWCA Civ 309, at [31]

[152] [1971] UKPC 33

[153] [2004] EWCA Civ 233

33.4 From a practical perspective, transparency is critical. Any legal advice must ordinarily be given in the presence of the parties.[154] Once advice is delivered, each party must be given the opportunity to endorse it, challenge it, or invite clarification. This moment should not be treated as a formality. Practitioners should consider carefully whether the advice accurately reflects the correct legal tests, the proper sequencing of decision-making, and the relevant burdens or evaluative thresholds. Where legal advice is given to a panel in private, the legal assessor must "as soon as practicable after the deliberations" inform the parties of the advice given and any question which prompted the advice.[155]

33.5 It is generally sensible for counsel to engage with the legal assessor in advance of final submissions to identify the legal directions that are likely to be required; to ensure that all the relevant authorities, statutory provisions and structured tests are considered before advice is formulated. Where complex or contested legal issues arise, early engagement of this kind can materially reduce the scope for later challenge.

33.6 Where the parties disagree as to how oral evidence came out, or where the parties' representatives' notes and recollections diverge, the legal assessor may be asked to assist by reference to their contemporaneous note. That note is not determinative and cannot replace a transcript of the proceedings. If disagreement cannot properly be resolved in that way, the only satisfactory course is to obtain and consult a transcript.

---

[154] *Nursing and Midwifery Order 2001 (Legal Assessors) Order of Council 2004*, SI 2004/1763, Rule 2

[155] *Nursing and Midwifery Order 2001 (Legal Assessors) Order of Council 2004*, SI 2004/1763, Rule 4(a)

34 Duty to give reasons

34.1 FTP panels are duty-bound to give reasons for their decisions. These will be provided in writing at the conclusion of the relevant decision making. By convention, practitioners may consent to written reasons being provided later where, for example, a preliminary application is decided in a manner anticipated by both sides. That convention does not displace the duty; practitioners may withhold such consent and require written reasons before proceeding.

34.2 Reasons must explain why the panel has reached its conclusions and must be sufficient to enable an appellate court to determine whether an error of law has occurred. The standard is one of adequacy, not exhaustiveness. The High Court does "not expect the same standards of literary expression as those found in perfectly polished judgments from the Supreme Court;"[156] "it is axiomatic that reasons for a decision will always be capable of having been better expressed."[157]

34.3 Panels are not required to address every submission or recite every piece of evidence; "the Tribunal is under no obligation to record in its reasons every point in favour of the [registrant] in the evidence it has heard and read".[158] A panel must "say enough to explain why it had reached the conclusion that the NMC had proved its case".[159] A failure to mention a particular item of evidence does not, without more, establish error. "It is

[156] *General Medical Council v Awan* [2020] EWHC 1553 (Admin), at [12]

[157] *Commissioner of Police of the Metropolis, R (On the Application of) v Police Misconduct Tribunal* [2025] EWHC 3110 (Admin), at [61]

[158] *Awan*, at [12]

[159] *Suddock v Nursing and Midwifery Council* [2015] EWHC 3612 (Admin), at [67]

trite law […] that a first instance decision-maker is not to be taken to have overlooked a particular piece of evidence, simply because it is not referred to in the decision."[160]

34.4 Reasons must, however, engage with the main issues. In *R (Smith) v General Teaching Council for England*,[161] the Court of Appeal recognised that published determinations are primarily informative and will not usually set out detailed factual backgrounds or matters such as remorse in depth. That observation does not dilute the duty to provide reasons, but it does underline that adequacy is judged in context, bearing in mind that the parties are already familiar with the evidence and submissions.

> Every Tribunal (including the PCC of the GMC) needs to ask itself the elementary questions: is what we have decided clear? Have we explained our decision and how we have reached it in such a way that the parties before us can understand clearly why they have won or why they have lost?[162]

34.5 Appellate courts will ordinarily proceed on the basis that a specialist tribunal has taken into account all material before it unless there is a compelling reason to conclude otherwise; that "decisions of specialist tribunals are not expected to be the product of elaborate legal drafting. Their decisions should be read as whole; and in assessing the reasons given, unless there is a compelling reason to the contrary, it is appropriate to take it

---

160 *Imani v General Dental Council* [2024] EWHC 132 (Admin), at [148]

161 [2007] EWCA Civ 1675, at [19]

162 *Phipps v General Medical Council* [2006] EWCA Civ 397, at [85]

that the Tribunal has fully taken into account all the evidence and submissions."[163]

34.6 Where panels occasionally fall into error is not through brevity of reasons, but through substituting assertion for analysis. Reasoning "merely a generalised assertion that erasure would be a disproportionate sanction and that the [practitioner's] conduct was not incompatible with his continued registration"[164] will not suffice. Such an approach fails to explain how seriousness had been assessed or why the chosen sanction met the statutory objectives. Similar deficiencies led to a successful PSA appeal in *Lingham*, where the court emphasised that careful analysis of what occurred, and of its significance and seriousness, "goes directly to public protection", and that, even if the outcome might have been open to the panel, the failure to expose its reasoning meant that it had not properly applied the Sanctions Guidance.[165]

34.7 As a matter of practice, practitioners should be alert to the wording of a determination when it is handed down. Where there appears to be a discrepancy between the panel's oral decision and the written reasons, an ambiguity in formulation, or a misstatement that may materially affect the decision, it is permissible to invite the panel to clarify or correct the wording at that stage. Timely challenges of this nature can avoid entrenched errors and may be critical in preserving or narrowing issues on any subsequent appeal.

---

[163] *Ali v Solicitors Regulation Authority* [2021] EWHC 2709 (Admin), at [94]

[164] *General Medical Council v Stone* [2017] EWHC 2534 (Admin), at [53]

[165] *Professional Standards Authority v General Medical Council & Lingham* [2023] EWHC 967 (Admin), at [73] – [74]

CHAPTER FIVE

THE CHRONOLOGY OF A CONCERN

35 Referrals

35.1 Most fitness to practise proceedings originate in a referral to the NMC by an employer, self-referral, the police, or occasionally a service user. The referral stage is jurisdictional rather than adjudicative. The NMC is not assessing guilt but whether the information disclosed is capable, if proved, of engaging a statutory ground under Article 22 of the Nursing and Midwifery Order 2001.

36 Screening

36.1 The initial assessment or screening stage is often decisive. At this point, the NMC considers whether to close the case or escalate it within the fitness to practise process. The regulator's published position is that its role is not to punish past conduct, but to assess whether there is evidence of an ongoing risk to public safety, public confidence, or professional standards that could require regulatory action. Screening therefore operates as a jurisdictional and proportionality filter, not a fact-finding exercise.

36.2 The NMC approaches screening on the assumption that registrants are generally safe and competent professionals, unless there is evidence of harm, recklessness, or a current risk requiring restriction. Not every concern raised about a registrant will justify regulatory intervention, and many matters are capable of being managed more appropriately by employers.

36.3 The screening team will inform a registrant when a complaint is made and afford an opportunity to make representations. For practitioners, this is the first substantive opportunity in the NMC framework to argue absence of impairment. Although no burden of proof formally arises, representations should focus on current fitness to practise, insight, remediation, and the absence of ongoing risk. It is well established that impairment is a forward-looking concept and that not every allegation of misconduct warrants regulatory adjudication.

36.4 Over-engagement with disputed factual minutiae at this stage is often counterproductive and risks strengthening an otherwise marginal case by diverting attention from the central screening question: whether regulatory action is presently required at all.

36.5 The average time between referral and screening decision is 24 weeks.[166]

37 Post-screening

37.1 Where a concern passes the screening stage, it will advance by referral as appropriate to either the case examiners to determine where there is a case to answer on fitness to practice,[167] or the investigating committee where the allegation relates to fraudulent entry on the register.[168] In both cases, notice of the referral and case details must be served on the registrant under the respective FTP rules relating to each.[169]

[166] Professional Standards Authority "*Periodic Review – Nursing and Midwifery Council 2023/2024*", at [15.7]

[167] FTP rule 2A(2)

[168] FTP rule 2A(1)

[169] FTP rule 6A; FTP rule 3

38 Investigation

38.1 Before case examiner stage, matters are sent to the NMC's investigation team for further investigation.[170] The investigation stage is invariably lengthy. Statistics published by the NMC in September 2025[171] suggest that 71.6% of cases now resolve within 15 months.

38.2 During the investigation, the NMC will obtain documents, records and information from employers and third parties, and may seek information from any person under Article 25(1). Investigators invariably obtain witness accounts. Practitioners should challenge investigative drift, disproportionate requests, or attempts to expand a discrete concern into a generalised inquiry into character or competence.

38.3 Throughout the investigation, the NMC must keep under review whether the statutory criteria for an interim order under Article 31 are met. Interim-order risk is therefore live for the duration of the investigation.

38.4 During the investigatory stage, registrants are invited to respond to allegations, evidence, and draft charges. There is no legal obligation to answer every question posed by the regulator, and there is no adverse inference regime equivalent to criminal proceedings. However, silence can be deployed against a registrant at later stages as an absence of insight or engagement. Further, a failure to mention salient points will limit the scope of the enquiry and deprive the registrant (and any later panel) of material relevant to the dispute, which may result in later

[170] FTP rule 2A(4); FTP rule 6B

[171] https://www.nmc.org.uk/news/news-and-updates/nmc-maintains-progress-in-timeliness-of-fitness-to-practise-casework/

delay. Practitioners must therefore exercise disciplined judgement.

38.5 Admissions should be precise and limited to what is properly conceded. Registrants are expected to engage with reasonable lines of enquiry and frequently find to their benefit that the NMC's ability to source evidence (particularly patient records) vastly exceeds that of any registrant.

39 Consensual disposal

39.1 Many registrants are keen to avoid contested hearings, the lengthy and career-altering delays which precede them, and the associated stressors of a long, drawn-out FTP process. Commonly, registrants will consider what if any options are available to dispose of a matter by consent.

39.2 Consensual disposal is a mechanism by which fitness to practise proceedings are resolved by agreement between the NMC and the registrant, subject always to approval by a panel. That panel's discretion is not fettered by the agreement, and retains full responsibility for determining impairment, sanction, and any interim order.

39.3 A consensual disposal may be pursued only where the allegation has properly reached the adjudicative stage. In practice, this requires either a case examiner decision that there is a case to answer. Consensual disposal is not available at the investigation stage, though indication of an intention to pursue consensual disposal may expedite the process.

39.4 The essential precondition is full admission. The registrant must admit the factual allegations relied upon and must admit that their fitness to practise is impaired. Allegations will not be withdrawn merely to secure agreement, though where particular factual particulars add nothing to overall seriousness or can be reformulated without undermining seriousness, some scope for amendment exists in practice. An admission of impairment is non-negotiable.

39.5 Where the parties reach provisional agreement, it must be reduced to writing and will ordinarily include the agreed facts, impairment, sanction, and any interim order considered necessary. That agreement is then placed before a panel, either at a meeting (without parties present) or at a hearing, though more frequently the former. The registrant may request a hearing.[172]

39.6 The panel is not a rubber stamp. It must satisfy itself that the agreed outcome properly protects the public, maintains public confidence, and upholds professional standards in accordance with the overarching objective.[173] The panel must consider the agreement as a whole, applying the Indicative Sanctions Guidance. If the panel considers the proposed outcome to be too lenient or too severe, it must raise its concerns with the parties before reaching a final decision.

39.7 Where a panel accepts the agreement, it will nonetheless announce findings of fact, impairment, and sanction, give reasons explaining why the outcome satisfies the public interest, and publish its decision subject to any direction for privacy.

39.8 Consensual disposal therefore results in a substantive regulatory outcome; it is not a private resolution save for cases heard in private for other reasons. For practitioners, consensual disposal requires careful scrutiny: disciplined admissions and realistic sanction analysis.

---

[172] FTP rule 10(2)(a)

[173] Article 3

Voluntary removal

39.9 Voluntary removal is a statutory mechanism permitting consensual removal from the register.[174] It is not an informal withdrawal from proceedings. Removal is not a unilateral act on the part of the registrant; it must be approved on application by the registrant to the registrar or, where the case has reached a hearing, the appropriate panel.

39.10 An application for voluntary removal may be made by a registrant before or during a fitness to practise hearing, though voluntary removal applications will not be considered until the conclusion of the investigation phase. Where an application is made during a hearing, the panel should not be informed of the application until a decision on impairment is made. Thereafter, the panel will determine the application and make a recommendation to the registrar.

39.11 Voluntary removal is permissible only where the registrant accepts the substance of the regulatory concern and provides evidence that they do not intend to continue practising. It is not available as a means of avoiding scrutiny while preserving the ability to return to practice. In practice, voluntary removal is therefore considered unavailable in cases where the registrant denies allegations and where appropriate concession cannot be agreed between the parties.

39.12 The public interest is the controlling consideration.[175] While voluntary removal provides immediate public protection by removing the registrant from practice, the public interest in publicly upholding and declaring proper standards is often

[174] Rule 14, *Nursing and Midwifery Council (Education, Registration and Registration Appeals) Rules 2004*, SI 2004/1767 ('Registration rules')

[175] Registration rule 14(2B)(iii)

weighty. Voluntary removal is therefore unlikely to be granted where allegations are of such seriousness that public confidence would be undermined by the absence of public adjudication.

39.13 Where voluntary removal is granted before a hearing, there will be no public determination of facts or impairment. Where it is granted following a panel recommendation, the panel's findings on impairment will ordinarily be published. In all cases, a registrant will be required to sign a declaration undertaking not to apply for readmission for a five-year period, and the fact of voluntary removal will be recorded on the register and may be disclosed to employers, regulators, and other relevant enquirers.

39.14 Importantly, voluntary removal does not extinguish the regulatory concern. Any future application for readmission will require the registrar to consider the original allegations and the circumstances in which voluntary removal was granted. Practitioners should therefore advise registrants that voluntary removal is not a mechanism by which to bypass regulatory scrutiny by taking a career break.

<u>Retirement</u>

39.15 Retirement from practice does not deprive the NMC of jurisdiction. Regulators are entitled to continue proceedings where necessary to protect the public or maintain confidence, even where the registrant states that they do not intend to return to practice.

39.16 Similarly, seeking to leave the profession by allowing registration to lapse either by declining to revalidation or pay fees will not have the effect of depriving the NMC of jurisdiction. That statutory scheme specifically provides that no registration may lapse where a registrant is subject to an allegation engaging Article 22,[176] or where a registrant is subject to interim or substantive conditions of practise or suspension.[177]

40 Case to answer

40.1 The investigation culminates procedurally in referral to the case examiners and the service of a notice of referral.[178] The notice to the registrant must be accompanied by all documents relating to the allegation which have not been disclosed previously.[179] This is often the registrant's first opportunity to see the whole evidential case, hence practitioners should scrutinise disclosure and raise any deficiencies immediately.

40.2 The notice must invite the registrant to make written representations, to be received within 28 days of the date of the notice.[180] It is generally unwise to treat representations at the case to answer stage as a forum for running the substantive defence. There is no obligation on the registrant to provide a full factual account. Representations should focus on matters material to the case to answer decision: prima facie case; absence of ongoing risk; remediation; insight; proportionality; and whether regulatory adjudication is required at all. Material volunteered at this stage will form part of the permanent evidential record and may be relied upon later by either party.

---

[176] Registration rule 14(4)(a)

[177] Registration rule 14(4)(b)

[178] FTP rule 6A

[179] FTP rule 6A(2)(a)

[180] FTP rule 6A(2)(b)

40.3 Upon expiry of the 28-day period, the matter is considered by two case examiners.[181] The Case Examiners must determine, on the material obtained by the Council and any representations made, whether there is a case to answer.[182] This is an evaluative decision taken on the papers. It is not a fact-finding exercise and does not involve resolving contested evidence.

40.4 Where the case examiners agree there is no case to answer, the case is closed. They may nonetheless issue advice or a warning to the registrant.[183] The parties must be notified of the decision.[184] A warning or advice shall take effect only after the expiry of the appeal period, or the disposal of any appeal where one is lodged.[185]

40.5 Where the case examiners agree that there is a case to answer, they must either refer the allegation to the fitness to practise committee or recommend undertakings,[186] unless they consider that there is a realistic prospect of a striking-off order, in which case undertakings are not available.[187]

40.6 Practitioners should direct representations at this stage to current fitness to practise, proportionality, and disposal. Even where referral is unavoidable, focused submissions at this stage can materially shape the scope and framing of the case that proceeds.

---

[181] FTP rule 6C

[182] FTP rule 6C(1)

[183] FTP rule 6C(2B)

[184] FTP rule 6C(3)

[185] Article 26(10)

[186] FTP rule 6C(2)

[187] FTP rule 6C(2A)

41 Undertakings

41.1 Where the case examiners agree that there is a case to answer, they may recommend that the matter be disposed of by way of undertakings agreed with the registrant, rather than referral to the Fitness to Practise Committee.

41.2 Undertakings are a consensual regulatory outcome. They have effect only if accepted by the registrant and approved in accordance with the rules. They may impose restrictions or requirements on the registrant's practice, including conditions analogous to conditions of practice orders, and may include requirements relating to supervision, training, health, or conduct. Their purpose is protective and remedial, not punitive.

41.3 Where undertakings are agreed, the allegation is not referred on, and no finding of impairment is made. The Registrar must notify the registrant and the person making the allegation of the outcome and reasons. Undertakings are time-limited and subject to monitoring. Breach of undertakings, or refusal to agree them, may result in referral of the allegation to the Fitness to Practise Committee.

41.4 For practitioners, undertakings provide a mechanism to resolve cases proportionately where risk can be managed without adjudication. Representations should focus on suitability, workability, and proportionality, and on why consensual disposal sufficiently protects the public and the wider public interest.

42 Preliminary FTP Meetings

42.1 Where a case to answer decision is given in the affirmative, the case proceeds to an FTP committee.

42.2 Preliminary meetings of the committees are a formal mechanism within the NMC FTP framework for resolving procedural and evidential issues in advance of the substantive hearing. Their purpose is case management in the true sense: to identify and determine matters which affect the scope, fairness, and efficient conduct of the final hearing, and to ensure that the panel charged with deciding the facts does so on a safe evidential footing.

42.3 Panels at preliminary meetings enjoy broad procedural powers to give "directions as to the conduct of the case and for the consequences of failure to comply with such directions."[188] A preliminary meeting may be convened at the request of a party or of the panel's own motion. It may take place remotely or in person, and may be conducted by the same panel that will later hear the case or by a differently constituted panel, depending on the circumstances and the nature of the issues to be determined. All preliminary meetings are heard in private session.[189]

42.4 In practice, preliminary meetings are particularly valuable where an issue is capable of shaping the hearing, or where leaving it to be dealt with at the outset of the substantive hearing would risk unfairness or inefficiency. They allow the panel to make reasoned decisions without the pressure of live evidence and without exposing the substantive tribunal to material that may later be ruled inadmissible.

42.5 Practitioners should expect to prepare for a preliminary meeting with the same care as for any other hearing. Where an application is contested or legally significant, it is good practice

---

[188] Article 32(3)

[189] FTP rule 18(2)(c)

to lodge a short skeleton argument in advance, identifying the issue, the relevant rules and case law, and the relief sought.

42.6 Certain categories of application are particularly well suited to determination at a preliminary meeting.

42.6.1 Hearsay admissibility is a paradigm example. Where the NMC seeks to rely on hearsay evidence, admissibility should be addressed before the final hearing wherever possible, particularly where the evidence is from a witness whose attendance could be secured were the application refused.

42.6.2 Disputes about admissibility more generally are often best resolved in advance. Early rulings reduce the risk of improper material influencing the substantive panel and avoid the need for repeated directions to disregard evidence once it has been seen.

42.6.3 Applications for special measures are commonly suitable for preliminary determination. These may include applications for evidence to be given remotely, behind screens, with the assistance of intermediaries, or with restrictions on questioning.[190]

42.6.4 Joinder and severance also go directly to the structure of the hearing and the panel's evaluative task, and neither are well suited to determination in the midst of the evidence.

42.6.5 Applications to amend allegations are frequently dealt with at preliminary meetings, particularly where amendments are substantial, introduce new factual bases, increase seriousness, or are prompted by

[190] FTP rule 23(3)

perceived weaknesses in the NMC's case. Late amendment is a recurrent feature of regulatory proceedings.

42.6.6 Other matters that may appropriately be dealt with at a preliminary meeting include applications relating to proceeding in absence, disclosure failures, timetabling, and the scope or sequencing of witnesses.

42.7 The unifying principles are procedural fairness and proportionality. If an issue has the potential to determine whether an allegation proceeds at all, to affect how evidence is given or tested, or to shape the evidential landscape against which the panel will make its findings, it is usually better raised and resolved at a preliminary meeting. Used properly, preliminary meetings ensure that FTP hearings are focused and fair.

43 Beyond the preliminary meeting

43.1 Following any preliminary meeting(s), and subject to hearings relating to interim orders, the matter then proceeds to the substantive FTP hearing.

43.2 Prior to that final hearing, the NMC will populate and serve a case management form ('CMF'). The CMF is a structured information-gathering document issued once a case is in the adjudication phase, designed to fix the practical and procedural shape of the proceedings. It requires the registrant to confirm contact and representation details, indicate whether they seek a (contested) hearing or a (uncontested, unattended) meeting of the relevant FTP committee (and whether virtual or in person), respond to the charges and impairment, identify what evidence is agreed or disputed, state which witnesses are required to attend and in what format, and flag any points of law or admissibility objections. It also captures the registrant's position on preliminary meetings and case conferences, explores alternative disposal routes such as consensual panel determination or agreed removal, and collects logistical information to enable listing, timetabling and reasonable adjustments.

43.3 Historically, the CMF was served after the NMC served on the registrant the totality of its PIW (post-investigation work). It served the purpose of providing a clear basis for listing decisions. In practice, it is now more commonly served after a case is listed. Nonetheless, practitioners should treat the CMF as a case-defining document: admissions, disputes, witness requirements, and evidential objections stated within it commonly shape directions, and the scope of the final hearing.

43.4 The securing of a listing is, in practice, often the point at which significant delay becomes apparent. Although the CMF is intended to enable efficient timetabling, the interval between completion of the form and the hearing dates subsequently fixed is frequently prolonged, and delays extending well beyond a year are not unusual. Practitioners should be alert to the impact of these delays and manage expectations accordingly.

43.5 Invariably once a case is listed, the NMC will subsequently arrange a case conference; a discussion between the responsible lawyer at the NMC and the registrant's representative. Case conferences are often productive and can serve to ensure that disclosure is complete and that allegations are sufficiently understood, with time estimates considered and deadlines agreed for the provision of further material or suggested redactions.

CHAPTER SIX

INTERIM ORDERS

44 **Purpose**

44.1 At any stage of the FTP process, the NMC may refer a case to a practice committee to consider an interim order restricting the registrant's practice.

44.2 Interim orders are a protective mechanism which functions to address identified risks pending determination of the substantive allegation. The power to impose an interim order derives from Article 31 of the Nursing and Midwifery Order 2001, and is given procedural effect by Part 3 of the FTP rules.

44.3 An interim order may be imposed only where it is necessary for the protection of members of the public, otherwise in the public interest, or in the interests of the registrant.[191] Interim orders are not justified merely because an allegation is serious, because an investigation is ongoing, or because public concern exists in the abstract. The inquiry is risk-based:

> "the focus of IOPs when determining an application for an interim order and the court when determining an extension application is on whether, in the light of the allegations made, an order is necessary for the protection of the public or is otherwise desirable and in the public interest, or in the interests of the practitioner concerned, with the onus being on the [regulator] to establish the necessity or desirability and the proportionality of making the order sought by the [regulator]. It is not an

---

[191] Article 31(2)

inquiry which is concerned with the truth or accuracy of the allegations made, which is a matter for the Fitness to Practise Panel in due course."[192]

45 Notice

45.1 Subject to limited exceptions, a Practice Committee may not make, vary, replace, confirm or revoke an interim order unless it is satisfied that an interim order notice has been served.[193]

45.2 The interim order notice must invite the registrant to attend the hearing, or to make written representations if they do not wish to attend, and must state why in the NMC's view an interim order may be necessary for public protection, the public interest, or the registrant's own interests. A notice that merely recites the statutory language without identifying the alleged risk will be inadequate.

45.3 Service must be effected within such time as is reasonable in all the circumstances.[194] What is reasonable depends on urgency, the nature of the alleged risk, and the practical ability of the registrant to respond.

46 Proceeding in absence

46.1 The Committee has the power to proceed in the absence of the registrant or in the absence of written representations,[195] but only where all reasonable efforts have been made to effect service, or the registrant has indicated that they do not wish to appear or be heard. These safeguards apply equally to review

[192] *Kakade v General Medical Council* [2013] EWHC 2110 (Admin), at [7]

[193] FTP rule 8(1)

[194] FTP rule 8(4)

[195] FTP rule 8(6)

hearings.[196] A failure to scrutinise service and engagement carefully risks procedural unfairness.

47 Thresholds for imposition

47.1 The necessity requirement is not a nicety. In recent years, the NMC has been criticised[197] by the courts for overlooking the centrality of the requirement:

> "It is not clear to me from this case and a series of other cases that the high bar imposed by the legislation before an interim order is made is, in practice, being generally applied, particularly in the context of cases that are taking far too long to resolve. An interim order should not be imposed because the Practice Committee have a concern that, if no order were to be made and there is a later patient safety incident, the NMC may be criticised.
>
> Whilst I accept that the Practice Committee have a difficult job in balancing risks, the Order sets a deliberately high test of necessity. An interim order can only be imposed if, on the evidence for that individual case, a strict test of necessity for the imposition of an interim orders is established. The "necessary" test means that the Practice Committee has to be satisfied to a civil standard that it is really necessary to impose the order for one of the stated purposes and, if some form of sanction meets the necessity test, that no lesser form of sanction can be justified. That is a higher test than it being

[196] FTP rule 8(7)

[197] *Nursing and Midwifery Council v Richmond* [2025] EWHC 1828 (Admin), at [23]

desirable for such an order to be made, albeit the test is not one as high as being absolutely essential.[198]

47.2 Where allegations are yet to be determined by an FTP panel, the NMC will have to satisfy the panel considering the interim order application that there is at least a *prima facie* case in respect of impairment on at least one statutory ground. If there is no such case, an order cannot be considered necessary to safeguard against any risk arising. This often results in interim order hearings involving submissions of the evidential strength of concerns which have not yet been investigated. It is a delicate act. As the courts have made clear, "an interim panel cannot and should not seek to decide the credibility or merits of a disputed allegation and at most can satisfy itself that there is a prima facie case that an allegation is well founded."[199] "That role is not to undertake the definitive examination of the allegations against the [registrant] or to decide on the fairness of the investigation,"[200] but to "satisfy itself that [...] there "may" be impairment of a practitioner's fitness to practise."[201]

47.3 In considering whether to impose an interim order, the panel must also undertake an assessment of proportionality, remaining aware that "the need to protect the public during the period before a competent investigation can be properly completed will often cause hardship and that sometimes that

---

198 *Nursing and Midwifery Council v Persand* [2023] EWHC 3356 (Admin), at [51] – [52]

199 *Aston v United Kingdom Council for Psychotherapy* [2025] EWHC 3288 (KB), at [78]

200 *Kumar v General Medical Council* [2013] EWHC 452 (Admin), at [27]

201 *Kumar*, at [27]

hardship, will in the end prove to have been unjustified because the allegations will not be proved":[202]

> The importance of the principle of proportionality in determining whether an interim order should be made pending the resolution of as yet unproven allegations faced by the practitioner, cannot be overstated. A suspension has potentially three very important consequences for a practitioner. First there is the impact upon the person's right to earn a living [...] Secondly, there is the obvious detriment to him in terms of his reputation. Thirdly it deprives the practitioner of showing that during the relevant period he has conducted himself well and competently and '*so, as it were, enhanced his prospects in front of the panel undertaking the final hearing*' (per Davis J. in *Sheikh* at paragraph 18)[203]

47.4 The statutory grounds (public protection; public interest; registrant's interests) are distinct and must be analysed separately.

47.4.1 Public protection requires evidence of a real risk of harm if the registrant were to practise unrestricted, though harm is interpreted widely; "to protect the public, to maintain public confidence in the [...] professional and to maintain high standards of behaviour by [...] practitioners. Each aspect of this threefold purpose must be properly considered for each secures the protection of the public."[204]

---

202 *Kumar*, at [39]

203 *Houshian v General Medical Council* [2012] EWHC 3458 (QB), at [13]

204 *Council for the Regulation of Health Care Professionals v General Dental Council* [2005] EWHC 87 (Admin), at [49]

47.4.2 Public interest is not a free-standing concept of reputational concern, but a narrow basis engaged only where interim restriction is necessary to maintain confidence in the profession pending resolution. "An order on public interest grounds is only justifiable in a relatively rare case,"[205] though "in considering whether the public interest calls for suspension (even before looking at proportionality) [it is] relevant to consider what the reaction of the public would be when the disciplinary process is complete and it is apparent that suspension did not occur."[206] The consideration is of "the likelihood of serious damage to public confidence in the profession if a registrant were allowed to continue to work with patients pending the resolution of unproved allegations against him".[207]

47.4.3 The registrant's own interests commonly arise in health cases, but do not permit paternalistic intervention absent necessity.

48 Types of interim order

48.1 The panel may impose an interim conditions of practice order or an interim suspension order.[208] Conditions must be preferred where they are capable of addressing the identified risk.

---

[205] *Persand*, at [22]

[206] *Harry v General Medical Council* [2012] EWHC 2762 (QB), at [16]

[207] *D v General Medical Council* [2015] EWHC 847 (Admin), at [24] (original emphasis)

[208] Article 31(2), *Nursing and Midwifery Order 2001*

48.2 The panel must consider whether workable, enforceable conditions could sufficiently mitigate risk before imposing suspension. There "should be no such thing as a "standard" set of conditions because the necessity test has to be satisfied with regard to each condition on the facts of each individual case before it can be lawfully imposed."[209] Conditions must not be formulated such that they operate in effect as a suspension.

48.3 Suspension is the most restrictive measure and must be justified by reference to necessity, not caution.

48.4 When a panel gives reasons for its decision, these must engage properly with proportionality. The High Court has criticised decisions which do "no more than state a conclusion that imposing conditions could not address the risks identified and that an interim suspension order is proportionate."[210]

49 Duration of order

49.1 The interim order powers of the NMC are capped; interim orders may be made for a maximum duration of 18 months.

49.2 Though in practice the NMC will invariably seek an interim order for the maximum permitted duration, citing the lengthy backlog of cases, "it should not be overlooked that Parliament has provided that 18 months is the maximum period of suspension that the Panel can impose. There will be many cases in which suspension is proportionate for a short period but not for as long as 18 months, given the very serious consequences it

[209] *Persand*, at [52]

[210] *MXM v General Medical Council* [2022] EWHC 817 (Admin), at [85]

has upon the doctor concerned. 18 months should not become a default position."[211]

50 Evidence and approach

50.1 Interim order decisions are made on incomplete material. Hearsay and preliminary evidence (such as referral forms) are admissible, but the weight attached to such material must reflect its provisional nature.

50.2 Panels must guard against making findings that trespass into the substantive determination.

50.3 Context, existing workplace restrictions, supervision, and employer action are all material to the assessment of necessity.

51 Reviews

51.1 Interim orders are subject to mandatory review. On review, a panel may confirm, revoke, vary or replace an interim order. A review is not a rehearing, but requires the panel to consider whether the order remains necessary and proportionate in light of any change in circumstances. The panel may receive any (new) evidence necessary to discharge its obligations.[212]

51.2 Progress of the investigation, compliance with conditions, remediation, and the passage of time are all relevant. The burden remains on the NMC to justify continuation of restriction.

[211] *Harry*, at [18]

[212] FTP rule 26(2)(a)

52 Appeals

52.1 There is a statutory right of appeal to the High Court. Common grounds include misapplication of the necessity test and failure to consider less restrictive alternatives.

53 Advocacy

53.1 Interim order hearings require disciplined advocacy. FTP rule 26 dictates the order to be followed: the NMC shall address the panel on necessity, type of order and length. The registrant then has an opportunity to respond and call evidence.[213]

53.2 Submissions should focus should be on necessity, proportionality, and present risk, not on rehearsing the substantive defence. Where conditions are viable, they should be proposed with precision. Concessions should be tactical and controlled.

53.3 Above all, practitioners should resist the normalisation of interim restriction as an automatic response to allegations and defaulting to an 18-month term without clear justification.

[213] FTP rule 26(2)(b)

CHAPTER SEVEN

THE SUBSTANTIVE FTP HEARING

54 Attendance

54.1 In recent years, remote hearings have become an established feature of the NMC's FTP process. Panels must be satisfied that a remote format permits effective participation by all parties, including the registrant, witnesses, and representatives. Considerations include the registrant's access to suitable technology, the ability to communicate privately with legal representatives, and the panel's capacity to observe witnesses giving evidence. The NMC has committed to keeping at least 50% of its hearings in person.

54.2 Remote attendance is by way of Microsoft Teams and is often appropriate where issues are narrow, evidence is largely documentary, or the registrant's circumstances make in-person attendance impracticable.

54.3 Hybrid hearings, in which some participants attend in person and others remotely, are common. In practice where a panel attends in-person, the case presenter and legal assessor will also do so. Remote participants join by Microsoft Teams, with a single camera covering the hearing room; it is invariably impossible when joining this way to see anything of substance. Though each panel member, the legal assessor and case presenter have separate microphones, the quality of audio is often troublesome. Given the technological limitations, practitioners should be alert to the risk that a registrant attending a hybrid hearing remotely may appear disengaged.

55 Transcription

55.1 The NMC is required to record all hearings in writing or electronic form.[214] The registrant has an absolute entitlement to the transcript.[215] Requests for transcripts are most commonly made where hearings are adjourned part-heard.

55.2 Practitioners in recent years have faced significant difficulty with the transcripts provided. Where, historically, proceedings would have been recorded and transcribed by a transcription company, the general approach now is to use the transcription function of Microsoft Teams. The quality of such transcripts is variable.

> "I was also provided with extracts of a sketchy transcript written by Microsoft Teams which is of some, but limited assistance."[216]

55.3 Where a hearing is plainly at risk of going part-heard, or more generally, practitioners should request that the audio from a hearing be recorded and made available separately.

56 Private/Public hearings

56.1 Subject to limited exceptions, FTP hearings must be conducted in public.[217] Private hearings mark a significant departure from the principle of open justice, which is "a fundamental principle of the common law [...] There are two particular aspects to the principle. The first is that the public should be free to attend

---

[214] FTP rule 27

[215] FTP rule 27(2)

[216] *Phillips v Nursing and Midwifery Council* [2025] EWHC 2993 (Admin), at [6]

[217] FTP rule 19(1)

court proceedings [...] The second aspect of open justice is that the proceedings are freely reportable."[218]

56.2 The public nature of hearings is itself a feature by which public confidence in the profession, and therefore the NMC's overarching objective,[219] can be maintained:

> "Public confidence in the profession and its reputation is [...] protected by hearings [...] being held in public. It not only ensures that matters are open to proper scrutiny such that the proper administration of justice in this domestic setting is done, but it enables the public to see what steps are taken to ensure that only those who it can properly be said have a suitable character are admitted into the profession."[220]

56.3 Where a hearing relates solely to an allegation concerning the registrant's physical or mental health, it must be held in private,[221] except where the provisions of FTP rule 19(2A) apply.

56.4 In all other cases, hearings may be held wholly or partly in private only where the panel is satisfied, that this is justified by the interests of a party, a third party (including a complainant, witness or patient), or the public interest, and that those interests outweigh the prejudice to open justice.[222]

---

218 *Solicitors Regulation Authority v Spector* [2016] EWHC 37 (Admin), at [19] – [20]

219 Article 4(4A)(b)

220 *L v The Law Society* [2008] EWCA Civ 811, at [41]

221 FTP rule 19(2)

222 FTP rule 19(4)

56.5 In practice, rule 19 applications commonly take the form of applications to hear the case in private session insofar as the medical history of individuals (patients or the registrant) or family circumstances are to be discussed. A proportionate balancing of Article 8 rights against the principle of open justice underpins the exercise.

56.6 All rule 19 applications are themselves heard in private session.[223] Panels must give reasons when returning a decision.

56.7 Where all or part of a hearing is heard in private, the public gallery is closed; a separate private version of any transcript commenced; and a separate private version of any determination will record those matters subject to the rule 19 direction. Parties will be expected to alert the panel if questions are about to be asked or answers given that stray into rule 19 protected territory, though where no observers are present the transcript can be amended retrospectively.

57 Panel Composition

57.1 Substantive fitness to practise hearings are determined by a panel. Panels are composed of a chair, a registrant member drawn from the same part of the register, and a lay member,[224] though the chair may satisfy the lay or registrant role.[225] This tripartite structure reflects the regulatory aim of combining professional insight, public perspective, and procedural oversight. It is not absolute, with a permissible quorum of two

---

[223] FTP rule 18(2)(c)

[224] *Nursing and Midwifery Council (Practice Committees) (Constitution) Rules 2008*, SI 2008/3148, Rule 6(10) (Constitution rules)

[225] Constitution rule 6(10)(c)

where "it is not reasonably practicable" to secure a three-person panel.[226]

57.2 The chair (usually addressed as "Sir" or "Madam;" occasionally "Chair") is responsible for managing the hearing and ensuring that proceedings remain fair, focused, and proportionate. While the chair may take a more active role in case management, they must not descend into advocacy.

57.3 The legal assessor, independent of the parties, advises the panel on matters of law, procedure, and regulatory principle. The assessor does not participate in fact-finding or decision-making, though will often accompany the panel in their deliberations.

58 Chronology of the Hearing

58.1 A substantive fitness to practise hearing ordinarily follows a recognisable sequence,[227] though panels may deviate from that sequence where they see fit. Deviations usually take the form of splitting stage 1 into separate deliberations and corresponding submissions on facts and grounds; or in cases where significant agreement is made, hearing stages together under the acknowledgement that the panel may disregard what it has heard in relation to later stages if, in its judgement, those stages are not reached.

58.2 Generally, the sequence matters. Panels should ordinarily resist the temptation to blur stages and never import considerations from later stages prematurely, particularly when determining facts or impairment.

---

[226] Constitution rule 6(11)

[227] FTP rule 24

59 Preliminary Applications

59.1 Preliminary applications set the procedural framework for the hearing and often shape its course. They are usually addressed at the outset, but applications may arise at any stage.

59.2 Common preliminary applications include applications for a hearing to proceed in private (a "rule 19 application"), applications to amend the charges, applications concerning the admission or exclusion of evidence, applications for special measures for witnesses, and applications to proceed in absence. Applications to amend the charges are particularly common at the preliminary stage.

59.3 Applications concerning witnesses often arise in cases involving vulnerable witnesses or sensitive subject matter. These may include applications for evidence to be given behind screens, by video-link, or with other protective measures. The panel must ensure that any such measures do not unduly restrict the registrant's ability to challenge the evidence and use of special measures requires a careful balancing exercise. The test is framed, however, as one of necessity.[228]

59.4 In determining any preliminary application, panels should give clear reasons.

59.5 From an advocacy perspective, preliminary applications are often the first opportunity to influence the tone of the hearing, to define the scope of the issues, and to ensure that the registrant is not placed at an unfair disadvantage. They should be prepared carefully and advanced with precision. It is often productive for the parties' representatives to discuss the nature of applications

[228] FTP rule 23(2)

to be made before the hearing to ensure that comprehensive advice can be given expeditiously.

60 Reading of the Charges and Pleas

60.1 At the commencement of the hearing, the registrant will be asked to confirm their name and NMC PIN number.[229] Where a registrant is not present, the NMC will address the panel on the steps taken to effect service of the notice of hearing and invite the panel to proceed in absence.

60.2 Thereafter, the substantive hearing formally begins with the reading of the charges.[230] The panel chair should ensure that the charges are read clearly and accurately.

60.3 The registrant is then invited to indicate whether the facts alleged are admitted or denied.[231] Some chairs prefer to have the charges read in full before asking this question; others prefer a response after each (sub)particular. Often, counsel will respond on behalf of the registrant to confirm whether an allegation is "admitted", "denied" or "admitted in part" (setting out succinctly any caveat to admission).

60.4 Where facts are admitted, these are announced as having been found proved by admission.[232]

60.5 Even where all facts are admitted, the panel must still determine whether those facts amount to misconduct or another statutory ground, and whether the registrant's fitness to practise is currently impaired. Although the chair may ask whether

[229] FTP rule 24(2)(a)

[230] FTP rule 24(2)(b)

[231] FTP rule 24(4)(a)

[232] FTP rule 24(5)

misconduct and impairment are admitted,[233] such admissions do not carry the same evidential consequence. An admission of facts does not equate to an admission of misconduct or impairment.

61 The NMC Opening

61.1 The regulator's opening serves a familiar purpose; to outline the case, identify the statutory grounds relied upon, and explain how the regulator says the evidence will establish those grounds and support a finding of impairment. Openings need not be comprehensive, but should be sufficiently detailed to accurately summarise the evidence as the regulator sees it.[234]

61.2 A proper opening should be measured and focused. It should identify the key allegations, summarise the evidence to be called, and highlight the issues likely to be contested. It should not amount to advocacy on sanction or stray into commentary on the registrant's character beyond that which is strictly relevant.

61.3 Where the opening raises issues of admissibility or scope that have not been addressed in preliminary applications, it may be appropriate to raise those matters at that stage rather than allowing them to persist throughout the hearing.

62 The NMC Case in Evidence

62.1 The regulator bears the burden of proving the facts alleged. Its case is ordinarily presented through witness evidence and documentary material.

---

233 FTP rule 24(4)(b)

234 *Webberley v General Medical Council* [2023] EWHC 734 (Admin), at [102] – [104]

62.2 Where facts are admitted, and where arranged in advance, the NMC may at this stage rely upon any statement of agreed facts. Where no such statement exists, the panel "should feel bold, where the facts have been opened only, (not canvassed thoroughly in evidence), to resolve any material issues they have by questioning as far as they need to do so, to clarify the central issues arising."[235]

62.3 Witnesses then give evidence on oath or affirmation.[236] Though the usual practice of asking a witness to confirm and adopt their statement as evidence-in-chief is permissible, particularly in cases where registrants attend unrepresented, panels tend to prefer a fuller examination-in-chief and may request that case presenter adopt such a course; to "go through the statement" with the witness.

62.4 Each witness may be cross-examined by the opposing party,[237] with the caveat that an alleged victim of sexual misconduct may not be cross-examined by an unrepresented registrant.[238]

62.5 Thereafter, the calling party may re-examine.[239] Re-examination is limited to matters arising from cross-examination. It should not be used to introduce new material.

62.6 Panels may then, and invariably do, ask questions of witnesses. Such questions should be neutral in tone. Panels must avoid assuming the role of advocate or giving the impression that they

---

[235] *Professional Standards Authority v General Medical Council & Lingham* [2023] EWHC 967 (Admin), at [79]

[236] FTP rule 22(1)

[237] FTP rule 22(3)(b)

[238] FTP rule 23(4)

[239] FTP rule 22(3)(c)

have reached a conclusion before hearing all the evidence. A panel member, when "forming an opinion as to the propriety or otherwise of what has been done or omitted to be done is entitled to a degree of latitude in the form and style of the questions which may be asked. The questions must of course be relevant to the issues before the inquiry."[240] "The members of the panel are not to be criticized for not asking questions in the way in which a professional advocate would."[241] Questions should focus on the matters to be decided, avoiding lines of questioning the "relevance of which [is] nil or so tenuous as to amount to vexing the witness rather than illuminating the factual issues."[242] Panels should ensure that questions are structured and not duplicative:

> The members of the panel asked the Appellant 44 questions in the course of 22 minutes. I remind myself that short questions and short answers can be exchanged quickly nonetheless this was not a case where there was a series of measured and structured questions with measured replies. Moreover, there is force in the Appellant's point that the panel members seem to have returned to the same topic at different times having given the impression that they had moved on from that issue and had been satisfied with the Appellant's answers.[243]

---

240 *Roylance v General Medical Council* [1999] UKPC 16, at [14]

241 *Nurrish v Nursing And Midwifery Council* [2026] EWHC 2 (Admin), at [67]

242 *Beard v General Osteopathic Council* [2019] EWHC 1561 (Admin), at [55]

243 *Nurrish v Nursing And Midwifery Council* [2026] EWHC 2 (Admin), at [66]

62.7 A witness of fact may not observe the hearing until the conclusion of their evidence.[244]

62.8 Documentary evidence often plays a significant role, particularly where contemporaneous clinical notes are available. Often, clinical records are included in the hearing bundle unexhibited. Though not impermissible, given the broad discretion to admit relevant evidence, practitioners often have to put records to witnesses who, until the day of the hearing, were unaware of them or have not had time to consider their content. Short adjournments for witnesses to familiarise themselves with documents are common.

63 Half-Time Submissions

63.1 At the close of the regulator's case, the registrant may make a submission that there is no case to answer.[245] A submission may be invited of the panel's own volition.[246] The *Galbraith* test applies:

> "(1) If there is no evidence that the crime alleged has been committed by the defendant there is no difficulty—the judge will stop the case.
>
> (2) The difficulty arises where there is some evidence but it is of a tenuous character, for example, because of inherent weakness or vagueness or because it is inconsistent with other evidence.
>
> (a) Where the judge concludes that the prosecution evidence, taken at its highest, is such that a jury properly

[244] FTP rule 22(6)

[245] FTP rule 24(7)

[246] FTP rule 24(7)(ii)

> directed could not properly convict on it, it is his duty, on a submission being made, to stop the case.
>
> (b) Where however the prosecution evidence is such that its strength or weakness depends on the view to be taken of a witness's reliability, or other matters which are generally speaking within the province of the jury and where on one possible view of the facts there is evidence on which the jury could properly come to the conclusion that the defendant is guilty, then the judge should allow the matter to be tried by the jury."[247]

63.2 A half-time submission can be made in respect of the facts,[248] or on the premise that even were the facts established (or where admitted), they could not amount to the statutory ground of impairment.[249]

63.3 Where an application is made, the registrant goes first; the NMC responds; the legal assessor reminds the panel of the test to be applied; and the panel retires to deliberate before returning with a decision. Often, where an application is refused, the panel will suggest providing their written reasons at a later stage in the interests of expedition.

64 The Registrant's Case

64.1 If the case proceeds beyond half-time, the registrant may give evidence and call witnesses.

64.2 The decision whether the registrant should give evidence, and if so how many times, is a significant one. Registrant evidence

---

[247] *R v Galbraith* [1981] 1 W.L.R 1039, at 1042B-E

[248] FTP rule 24(7)

[249] FTP rule 24(8)

may be relevant to all three core questions the panel must determine: the facts, whether those facts amount to the statutory ground, and whether the registrant's fitness to practise is currently impaired. A registrant may give evidence at the factual stage, the impairment stage, both, or neither. Evidence at stage 1 may assist in contesting disputed facts or providing context, but it exposes the registrant to cross-examination. Evidence at stage 2 is directed not to what happened, but to insight, remediation, and the risk of repetition, and can therefore be influential on impairment even where facts or misconduct are admitted or found proved. In some cases, particularly where the factual matrix is largely documentary or admitted, it may be tactically preferable for the registrant to remain silent at stage 1 and give focused evidence only at the impairment stage. The choice requires careful assessment of the pleaded case and the risks inherent in cross-examination at each stage.

64.3 Where a registrant gives evidence only once, most commonly at the factual stage, and addresses matters relating to later stages, the panel should be directed to consider the evidence only for the purposes of the stage then under consideration, and to disregard any elements that are not yet relevant. Evidence touching on insight, remediation, or future risk may therefore be heard at stage 1 but put to one side, to be returned to (and relied upon) later.

64.4 The same order applies to registrant evidence:[250] examination-in-chief under oath or affirmation; cross-examination by the NMC; re-examination; panel questions; any questions arising from panel questions.

[250] FTP rule 22

64.5 Though uncommon, a registrant may opt to give an unsworn statement in evidence. There is no right to cross-examine on such a statement, nor is the panel entitled to ask questions. Accordingly, unsworn statements carry significantly less weight than evidence on oath or affirmation.

64.6 The registrant, if they are giving evidence, must do so before any defence witnesses are called. Supporting witnesses often include colleagues, supervisors, or experts. Their evidence must be relevant to the matters in issue and should not be used simply to bolster the registrant's character unless character evidence is properly admissible at that stage. Character evidence may be relevant where credibility is in issue or where the registrant's past conduct is relied upon as indicative of current impairment.

64.7 A person accompanying the registrant at the hearing, such as a union representative, may not be called as a witness.[251]

65 Closing Submissions

65.1 Closing submissions on the facts should identify the findings that the panel is invited to make and explain why those findings are or not supported by the evidence. Submissions should distinguish clearly between disputed and undisputed matters and should address credibility, reliability, and consistency where relevant.

65.2 Where dishonesty is alleged, the correct approach is that articulated in *Ivey v Genting Casinos (UK) Ltd.*[252] The fact-finding exercise requires the panel first to determine, on the balance of probabilities, the registrant's actual state of knowledge or belief as to the relevant facts. Once that is

---

[251] FTP rule 20(4)

[252] [2017] UKSC 67

established, the question of dishonesty is an objective one: whether the conduct was dishonest by the standards of ordinary decent people. Submissions should not elide these two conceptually distinct stages. There is no requirement that the registrant appreciated that their conduct would be regarded as dishonest,[253] nor any reverse burden to prove dishonest intent.[254]

65.3 Allegations pleaded in terms of a "failure to" do something necessarily imply the existence of a specific obligation said to have been owed by the registrant at the material time. Submissions should not ignore that, as a matter of proper factual analysis, the obligation is a condition precedent to any finding that the allegation is proved. The panel must therefore identify, with precision, the source and content of the alleged duty, whether arising from statute, contractual role, professional standards, local policy, or a specific instruction, and must be satisfied that the obligation applied to the registrant in the circumstances alleged. Absent clear proof of the obligation itself, an allegation framed as a "failure to" cannot be made out, regardless of whether the outcome is said to be undesirable or whether alternative steps might, with hindsight, have been preferable.

65.4 Where an allegation pleads conduct as being "sexual", submissions should address the test in s.78 Sexual Offences Act 2003 and the exemption in s.3.[255]

65.5 Where, however conduct is allegedly "sexually motivated", the test to be addressed in submissions on facts is whether "the

[253] *Ivey*, at [74]

[254] *Mobasseri v General Dental Council* [2025] EWHC 3006 (Admin), at [92] – [96]

[255] *General Medical Council v Haris* [2020] EWHC 2518 (Admin), at [57]ff

conduct was done either in pursuit of sexual gratification or in pursuit of a future sexual relationship."[256] The two are not "hermetically sealed alternatives,"[257] and such a pursuit on the part of a registrant need only "be a factor in the [conduct], not its 'but for' cause, for the allegation of sexual motivation to be made out."[258]

65.6 Closing submissions can be delivered orally or in writing. In practice, panels prefer written closings in complicated cases but are deterred from inviting them; there is no rule applicable to the form. Written closings may be adopted without reading into the record.

65.7 Where facts are admitted, submissions may focus on the proper characterisation of those facts and invite any findings beyond the allegations necessary to contextualise the conduct. An admission does not determine whether conduct amounts to misconduct or whether impairment is established, hence submissions around the facts at this stage may be useful.

65.8 Unless the panel has directed otherwise,[259] submissions should also address at this stage whether any combination of facts proven could amount to the statutory ground. Personal mitigation is generally irrelevant to this consideration.[260]

---

[256] *Basson v General Medical Council* [2018] EWHC 505 (Admin), at [14]

[257] *Haddon v United Kingdom Council for Psychotherapy* [2025] EWHC 1628 (KB), at [93]

[258] *Haddon*, at [89]

[259] FTP rule 24(1)

[260] *Campbell, R (On the Application of) v General Medical Council* [2005] EWCA Civ 250, at [46]

66 Legal advice

66.1 Before the panel retires to decide the facts and grounds, they must receive legal advice from the legal assessor. Legal advice will address the law as it relates to the stage in issue, the approach to be undertaken, and ordinarily reiterates the duty to give reasons. Legal advice shall be given in the presence of the parties.[261] Once advice is delivered, each party must be given the opportunity to endorse it, challenge it, or invite clarification. Where legal advice is given to a panel in private, the legal assessor must "as soon as practicable after the deliberations" inform the parties of the advice given and any question which prompted the advice.[262]

67 Decisions

67.1 Upon completion of their deliberations, and the drafting of written reasons, the panel returns to deliver their decision on the particular stage. In practice, the drafting process is often lengthy. Where facts or grounds are not established, the case ends. Where the case is to proceed, parties will be given an opportunity to read the decision before proceeding.

68 Stage 2 – Impairment

68.1 If the panel finds any ground established, the hearing proceeds to impairment. Both the NMC and the registrant may call further evidence at this stage. The order in which evidence is called mirrors that of stage 1.

---

[261] *Nursing and Midwifery Order 2001 (Legal Assessors) Order of Council 2004*, SI 2004/1763, Rule 2

[262] *Nursing and Midwifery Order 2001 (Legal Assessors) Order of Council 2004*, SI 2004/1763, Rule 4(a)

68.2 Submissions on impairment should be analytically distinct from submissions on facts. The question is not whether the conduct occurred, but whether the registrant's fitness to practise is currently impaired. Submissions should address both the personal and public components: the registrant's insight, remediation, and risk of repetition; and the need to maintain confidence in the profession and to uphold professional standards.

68.3 It is a common error to treat impairment as a retrospective assessment of wrongdoing. Submissions should emphasise that impairment is a forward-looking judgement, concerned with current risk and public confidence at the time of the hearing.

68.4 Where impairment is contested, submissions should engage with the evidence relied upon to demonstrate insight and remediation. Panels are assisted by concrete examples rather than general assertions of learning or regret.

68.5 Submissions should avoid straying prematurely into sanction. Panels must first determine whether impairment is established before considering outcome.

68.6 Again, the panel will receive legal advice in the traditional way, retire to consider their decision, and return with their written reasons.

69 Stage 3 – Sanction

69.1 If the panel finds that the registrant's fitness to practise is impaired, it must proceed to consider sanction. The purpose of sanction is protective. It is not to punish the registrant, but to protect the public, maintain confidence in the profession, and uphold proper professional standards.

69.2 The NMC may, at this stage, adduce evidence inadmissible at earlier stages, such as evidence of previous FTP decisions, or the extent of (non)compliance with interim conditions of practice.[263]

69.3 Sanction is an evaluative exercise in which the panel must identify the least restrictive outcome that adequately meets the regulatory objectives, giving appropriate deference to the Indicative Sanctions Guidance and explaining how it has informed the decision. The panel should work through the available sanctions in ascending order of seriousness, giving reasons where lesser outcomes are rejected, and must identify and weigh relevant aggravating and mitigating factors, guarding against sanction drift by focusing on current impairment rather than the historic seriousness of the conduct alone.

69.4 Submissions on sanction should be structured and proportionate, addressing how each sanction might strike a balance between interests, and how any proposed conditions would operate in practice.

69.5 Following legal advice, the panel will retire to make its decision. The final decision must be clearly reasoned to demonstrate proper engagement with the registrant's circumstances, the nature of the impairment, and the regulatory objectives, failing which it may be vulnerable to challenge. The decision will be announced on the panel's return.[264]

[263] FTP rule 24(13)(c)

[264] FTP rule 24(13)(a)

70 Interim Orders Following Determination

70.1 A substantive sanction does not take effect until 28 days after the notice of decision is sent.[265] Where an appeal is lodged within that period, the sanction is stayed pending determination of the appeal.[266]

70.2 The panel must therefore consider, in every case in which a sanction of conditions or suspension is imposed,[267] whether an interim order is required to cover the appeal period. Though not covered by rule 13(f), the power extends to and is most frequently used in cases of strike-off.[268]

70.3 Before making an interim order, the chair must invite submissions,[269] with the case presenter heard first and the registrant in reply. The panel must take those submissions into account,[270] obtain any relevant advice from the legal assessor, and afford the parties an opportunity to comment on that advice. The panel then deliberates in private, before returning with its decision.

70.4 The statutory tests for an interim order following determination mirror those applicable earlier in proceedings. Any interim order imposed must be time-limited and reasoned. Panels should explain why lesser measures are insufficient. Any interim order imposed should be consistent with, and not more

---

[265] Article 29(11)(a)

[266] Article 29(11)(b)

[267] FTP rule 13(f)

[268] Article 31(1)(c); Article 31(2)

[269] FTP rule 14(a)

[270] FTP rule 14(b)

restrictive than, the substantive order unless justified by necessity.

70.5 Often, consideration of an interim order after the handing down of a substantive sanction appears to involve a shorter deliberation, with panels returning quickly having given the matter consideration prior to receiving submissions. This stage should not be treated as an administrative addendum, but is a distinct consideration in its own right. The High Court has excoriated insufficiently reasoned interim order decisions:

> In addition to imposing a substantive sanction of 6-months suspension, the Panel also made an interim suspension order of 18-months' duration "in order to cover any appeal period". The consequence of that interim suspension order is that the Appellant has now been suspended from practising as a nurse for the past 13 months, and thus potentially for considerably longer that the total suspension period she might have served had she not appealed. [...] I think it right, however, to record my concern as to the lack of substantive reasoning provided by the Panel for imposing the interim order. No interim order had been made for restricting the Appellant's practise during the long period over which the FtP proceedings had been drawn out, prior to the Panel's decision.[...] Against this background, it is very difficult to understand why the Panel considered an interim suspension order to be "necessary for the protection of the public" and "otherwise in the public interest", as the relevant section of its Reasons asserted it to be. The Panel's reasoning (such as it was) evinces no consideration of the severity of the potential impact on the Appellant of an 18-month interim suspension order, its intrinsic potential to disincentivise her from appealing, or the risk of unfairness if her appeal ultimately succeeded but she had, in the meantime, been suspended from

> practising for a prolonged period. Those considerations ought, in my view, to be expressly thought about, and carefully weighed, by a Panel when it is considering whether to impose an interim suspension order. The Panel should also be clear as to the nature of the harm it fears could occur, absent the contemplated interim suspension order. Absent such careful weighing of the competing interests at play, it is hard to see how a Panel could properly decide that the imposition of an interim order was necessary and proportionate.[271]

71 Part-Heard Hearings

71.1 FTP hearings frequently adjourn part-heard due to time pressure, witness availability, illness, or other unforeseen disruption. Where this occurs, the immediate practical focus is on how the case will be resumed. Parties will usually be asked during the hearing to provide dates to avoid, with a firm preference that the hearing concludes with proposed dates agreed in principle and passed to the scheduling team. The panel itself has no listing function and cannot fix relisting dates.

71.2 Directions should ordinarily be given for the preparation and provision of transcripts in advance of the resumption, and in cases where outstanding legal arguments remain, it may be appropriate to list a short preliminary hearing before the resumed substantive hearing. Where a case adjourns part-heard with the panel in retirement, it is common for "panel days" to be scheduled ahead of resumption for private deliberation to continue.

[271] *Hindle v Nursing and Midwifery Council* [2025] EWHC 373 (Admin), at [120] – [122]

71.3 Practitioners should note that relisted hearings are often arranged in multiple shorter blocks because of availability constraints.

CHAPTER EIGHT

COMMON PROCEDURAL ISSUES

72 Case Management

72.1 The NMC's committees do not possess inherent jurisdiction.[272] Panels are statutory decision-makers whose powers are confined by the enabling legislation, though the absence of inherent jurisdiction does not render hearings procedurally rigid. The FTP rules[273] prescribe core procedural requirements while conferring broad discretion on panels to manage hearings fairly and effectively, including in circumstances not exhaustively anticipated by the rules:

> Rule 12 requires the Committee to conduct a hearing in accordance with the procedure set out in Part 5 of the Rules [...] Rule 24 of the Rules requires the Committee 'unless it determines otherwise' to conduct the initial hearing of an allegation 'in the following stages'. [...] Some of the components of those stages are mandatory ('shall') and some discretionary ('may').[274]
>
> [Rule] 24(1) gives the Committee power to decide, in an appropriate case, not to conduct a hearing in accordance

---

[272] *B, R (on the application of) v Nursing and Midwifery Council* [2012] EWHC 1264 (Admin), at [32]

[273] *The Nursing and Midwifery Council (Fitness to Practise) Rules 2004* (SI 2004/1761)

[274] *Professional Standards Authority v General Medical Council & Lingham* [2023] EWHC 967 (Admin), at [55]

> with the stages set out in rule 24 [but] that general power cannot be used to contradict the effect of the specific provisions in rule 24(6), (7) and (8).[275]

72.2 The panel's approach to procedural issues is informed by balancing two principal considerations reflected throughout the FtP rules: the interests of and fairness to the registrant;[276] and the public interest in promoting and maintaining public confidence in the professions and declaring and upholding proper standards,[277] both potentially being served by the "fair, economical, expeditious and efficient disposal of allegations."[278]

72.3 In practice, panels therefore ask whether the proposed course is authorised by an express rule, or if not expressly regulated, whether it is a lawful exercise of discretion consistent with the rules and the overarching objective.

73 Adjournments

73.1 FTP panels have a discretionary power to adjourn,[279] exercisable on application by the parties or of own the panel's own motion.[280] There is no presumption in favour of expedition or delay within the rules, which set express

---

[275] *Lingham*, at [57]

[276] Article 3(5)(ii)

[277] Article 3(4A)

[278] *General Medical Council v Adeogba* [2016] EWCA Civ 162 , at [17]

[279] FTP rule 32

[280] FTP rule 32(1)

requirements of fairness to the parties,[281] and the registrant individually.[282]

> "Where there is good reason not to proceed, the case should be adjourned; where there is not, however, it is only right that it should proceed."[283]

73.2 The exercise of the discretion is informed by general principles applicable elsewhere, including those articulated in *Jones*[284] and *Picton*,[285] noting that "the analogy between criminal prosecution and regulatory proceedings could not be taken too far given the important regulatory objective in play."[286] The seminal authority in the FTP sphere is *General Medical Council v Adeogba*.[287]

73.3 The central question is whether refusing or granting an adjournment would cause injustice.[288] Injustice is not equated with inconvenience or tactical disadvantage. The inquiry is whether the conduct of the hearing would be rendered unfair, having regard to the ability of the parties to participate effectively, test evidence, and present their case. "The principle

---

[281] FTP rule 32(2)(a)

[282] FTP rule 32(4)(c)

[283] *General Medical Council v Adeogba* [2016] EWCA Civ 162, at [19]

[284] *R v Jones (Anthony)* [2002] UKHL 5

[285] *Crown Prosecution Service v Picton* [2006] EWHC 1108 (Admin)

[286] *Sanusi v General Medical Council* [2019] EWCA Civ 1172, at [65]

[287] [2016] EWCA Civ 162

[288] FTP rule 32(2)(a)

of fairness also requires fairness to the regulatory body, witnesses and the public."[289]

73.4 Where adjournment is sought on medical grounds, the burden lies firmly on the registrant to provide cogent, specific medical evidence demonstrating unfitness to participate in the hearing, not merely unfitness to work.[290]

73.5 Submissions seeking an adjournment should be structured forensically toward the criteria in rule 32(4), rather than appealing to sympathy or convenience. The starting point is to identify with precision the unfairness said to arise if the hearing proceeds as listed; how that unfairness bears on the applicant party's ability to participate effectively or present their case; and whether "arrangements might be made short of an adjournment to accommodate the parties' difficulties."[291] It is often wise, within this exercise, to address in detail why the difficulty has arisen by reference to the chronology of the case and the history of correspondence between registrant and regulator (where necessary) as, in practice, panels are acutely sensitive to delay caused by lack of preparation or perceived tactical manoeuvring.

73.6 Submissions should also confront the countervailing public interest in expedition and finality, addressing why the prayed injustice in refusing adjournment outweighs the prejudice caused by delay. Where possible, submissions should identify the precise length of the adjournment sought and what steps will be taken during that period, so as to demonstrate that the proposed adjournment is a proportionate, targeted and time-

[289] *Tsolo v Nursing and Midwifery Council* [2025] EWHC 2324 (Admin), at [89]

[290] *General Medical Council v Hayat* [2018] EWCA Civ 2796, at [48]

[291] *Webberley v General Medical Council* [2022] EWHC 3520 (Admin), at [8]

limited means of curing the identified injustice rather than an open-ended delay.

73.7 Where proceedings other than interim order proceedings are adjourned, the panel must consider whether or not to make an interim order.[292] The NMC must then notify the parties as soon as practicable of the date, time and venue of the resumed hearing.[293] Panels should therefore anticipate, at the point of adjournment, the practical consequences for listing, continuity, and the availability of witnesses and representatives.

74 Joinder and severance

74.1 FTP rule 29 provides an express power of joinder. Joinder of allegations relating to two or more registrants arising from the same circumstances is permissible unless the panel is of the view that there is a risk of prejudice to the fairness of the proceedings.[294]

74.2 FTP rule 29(2) addresses joinder of categories of allegation against a single registrant. It permits multiple allegations to be heard together, but imposes a mandatory sequencing safeguard: an allegation relating to a conviction or caution must be heard after any allegation of misconduct has been heard *and* determined.

74.3 FTP rule 29(3) permits late joinder of a new allegation that is similar in kind or founded on the same facts as an existing referral, even where it is not contained in the original notice of hearing. The registrant must be informed of the new allegation and afforded a meaningful opportunity to make written

[292] FTP rule 32(5)

[293] FTP rule 32(3)

FTP rule 29(1)

representations, ordinarily within 28 days. Failure to respect those safeguards will undermine the fairness of any joined hearing.

74.4 The FTP rules contain no express provision for severance. In practice, any application to sever must therefore be framed by reference to FTP rule 29 itself, and in particular the threshold question of prejudice to the fairness of the proceedings.

74.5 In exercising these powers, panels should give clear, reasoned decisions explaining why joinder serves fairness, proportionality, and the statutory purpose of regulation. Reasons should address not only efficiency and expedition, but the registrant's right to a fair hearing and the integrity of the process. A failure to grapple with the prejudice caused by joinder, or to explain why severance is unnecessary, may itself give rise to appealable error.

75 Absent Registrant

75.1 Proceedings in the absence of the registrant represent a significant departure from the ordinary course of a fitness to practise hearing. The discretion to proceed in absence, although clearly within a panel's gift,[295] is "severely constrained"[296] and must be exercised with caution.

75.2 Where the registrant fails to attend and is not represented, the panel must first require the case presenter to adduce evidence that all reasonable efforts have been made, to serve the notice of hearing.[297] Proof of service is a necessary, but not sufficient, condition. Reasonable efforts will include service upon the

[295] FTP rule 21; FTP rule 8(6)

[296] *Tait v Royal College of Veterinary Surgeons* [2003] UKPC 34, at [8]

[297] FTP rule 21(2)(a)

address the registrant has given the NMC, whether that remains current or not.[298]

75.3 If satisfied that the notice of hearing has been duly served, the panel may either direct that the allegation be heard and determined notwithstanding the registrant's absence, or adjourn the hearing and issue directions.[299]

75.4 In line with some of the criminal authorities,[300] before deciding to proceed, the panel must consider whether the registrant's absence is voluntary, deliberate, or unexplained. Relevant factors include the registrant's prior engagement with the proceedings, any explanation advanced for the absence, and any evidence of illness, misunderstanding, or practical impediment. Even where voluntary absence is established, the panel must go on to consider whether it is fair and in the public interest to proceed. Relevant considerations include the likely length of any adjournment, the availability of and impact upon witnesses, the likelihood that an adjournment would secure attendance, and the potential prejudice to the registrant.

75.5 The modern approach to proceeding in absence was clarified by the Court of Appeal in *General Medical Council v Adeogba.*[301] While accepting that the principles in the criminal authorities provide "a useful starting point,"[302] the Court emphasised that regulatory proceedings are not criminal trials and must be approached in their own statutory context. The decision must be guided "by the main statutory objective of the

[298] *Jatta v Nursing and Midwifery Council* [2009] EWCA Civ 824, at [31]

[299] FTP rule 21(2)(a)-(b)

[300] Principally, *R v Jones (Anthony)* [2002] UKHL 5

[301] [2016] EWCA Civ 162

[302] *Adeogba*, at [17]

[regulator],"[303] and by the need for the "fair, economical, expeditious and efficient disposal of allegations."[304]

75.6 Fairness "fully encompasses fairness to the affected medical practitioner (a feature of prime importance)"[305] but it also includes fairness to the regulator and to the wider public interest. The Court warned against taking the criminal analogy too far, noting that regulators have no coercive powers to secure attendance and that it would "run entirely counter to the protection, promotion and maintenance of the health and safety of the public if a practitioner could effectively frustrate the process"[306] by deliberate non-engagement. "Where there is good reason not to proceed, the case should be adjourned; where there is not, however, it is only right that it should proceed."[307] The Court in *Adeogba* further underlined that professionals subject to regulation bear "a burden [...] to engage with the regulator"[308] as part of the responsibility assumed on admission to the profession.

75.7 The decision to proceed in absence must be reasoned and kept under review as the hearing progresses. However, where a registrant has chosen not to attend, and adverse findings made, "there is no general obligation on the [...] Tribunal to adjourn

[303] *Adeogba*, at [17]

[304] *Adeogba*, at [17]

[305] *Adeogba*, at [18]

[306] *Adeogba*, at [19]

[307] *Adeogba*, at [19]

[308] *Adeogba*, at [20]

or to provide a registrant with the opportunity to make submissions in mitigation of sanction."[309]

75.8 Panels must ensure that the proceedings remain fair notwithstanding the registrant's absence. While the regulator remains under a duty of fairness in presenting its case, the registrant's non-participation does not impose an obligation on the panel to compensate for tactical or voluntary disengagement. Where a registrant disengages from the process, the NMC "does not have to guess what the practitioner wants to put before the FTPP for the final hearing. Nor does the NMC have to sift through the historic case correspondence or the historic documents previously sent by the practitioner during, for instance, the interim suspension hearings and appeals from interim orders, to construct evidence files which the practitioner himself has not identified."[310] However, the NMC "should take reasonable steps to ensure that all relevant mitigation material provided by an absent registrant is available for consideration by the panel when it comes to deal with sanction. [...] That obligation extends only to reasonable searches for material that is objectively viewed as relevant. It must not be forgotten that [registrants] have their own obligations [...] to cooperate with their regulator."[311]

76 Absent Witness

76.1 Where a witness scheduled to give live evidence is not present or disengages, the panel must decide how the proceedings can continue fairly. The available options are practical, as no FTP

[309] *Sanusi v General Medical Council* [2019] EWCA Civ 1172, at [68]

[310] *Golden v Nursing and Midwifery Council* [2023] EWHC 619 (Admin), at [25]

[311] *Sanusi v General Medical Council* [2019] EWCA Civ 1172, at [84]

rule specifically envisages this situation, which in practice arises with surprising frequency.

76.2 The panel may adjourn to secure attendance under its adjournment discretion,[312] particularly where the evidence is central and the absence appears temporary or remediable. The panel may also explore whether arrangements would enable the witness to give evidence, including remote attendance, adjustments to questioning, or other procedural accommodations. Such measures are permissible outwith the vulnerable witness framework of rule 23; a "case management decision [...] deciding how evidence should be given."[313]

76.3 If attendance cannot be secured, the panel may be invited to admit the evidence in hearsay form. Alternatively, the opposing party may apply under rule 31 to exclude the evidence as unfair, especially where the inability to test it causes prejudice.

76.4 A distinction should be drawn between a witness who is entirely absent and one who attends but refuses to complete their evidence. Where a witness disengages mid-way, particularly during cross-examination or before panel questioning, fairness concerns abound. In such cases, the panel should consider whether reliance on the evidence is sustainable at all; whether it ought to be excluded.[314] If the evidence is not excluded, the panel must grapple in any later written reasons with the consequences of incomplete testing, which may justify attaching very limited, or no, weight to the evidence.

---

[312] FTP rule 32

[313] *Levett, R (On the Application Of) v Health and Care Professions Council* [2013] EWHC 3330 (Admin), at [27]

[314] *Freeman v General Medical Council* [2023] EWHC 45 (Admin), at [45]ff

76.5 In every case, the panel should identify why the witness is absent or disengaged, assess the importance of the evidence, and consider whether the resulting prejudice can realistically be cured by any procedural step short of exclusion. The overarching objective continues to apply, but does not displace the need for a fair hearing. Clear reasons should be given for the course adopted, particularly where evidence is retained despite one party being denied a proper opportunity to test it.

77 Absent Panel Member

77.1 In a part-heard case, any proposal to reconstitute the panel engages significant fairness considerations, particularly where oral evidence has already been heard or credibility assessments have been made. Although reconstitution is permitted, the panel must consider whether continuation before a differently constituted panel would be unfair, or whether fairness requires the hearing to recommence.

77.2 Where an ordinary panel member becomes unavailable during proceedings, the panel may not continue unless it remains properly constituted in accordance with the Committee Constitution Rules. If quorum of three is lost, the hearing shall ordinarily be adjourned if that panel member is to continue, though a panel may continue with a quorum of two.[315]

77.3 Though the FTP and Committee Constitution rules are silent on point, the courts have interpreted the analogous GMC scheme (similarly silent) as conferring a power to substitute in a new panel member at any stage:

> "the membership of the panel shall comprise medical and lay panellists selected by the Registrar. That power is not

[315] *Nursing and Midwifery Council (Practice Committees) (Constitution) Rules 2008*, SI 2008/3148, Rule 6(11)

expressly limited to the appointment of a panel at the outset of proceedings. On its face the power is not limited and could in principle be used to appoint panel members at any time. Furthermore it is in the interests of practicality and the proper administration of these disciplinary proceedings that there should be no limitation in principle to that power. It is of considerable importance that if indeed the panel is potentially liable to be inquorate, either because of unavailability or ineligibility, that the Registrar should have the power to appoint a substitute."[316]

77.4 The unavailability of the chair raises particular difficulty, given the chair's role in case management, procedural rulings, and control of the hearing. Substitution of the chair part-heard will often raise more serious fairness concerns than the loss of an ordinary panel member. Where the chair becomes unavailable, the remaining panel members must consider with particular care whether continuation before a new chair is appointed is fair. They may do so as a quorum of two, and may continue without a chair only where it is not "reasonably practicable" to secure a new chair.[317]

77.5 As with any decision to proceed following a change in constitution, the panel must invite submissions and give fully reasoned decisions.

[316] *Michalak, R (on the application of) v General Medical Council* [2011] EWHC 2307 (Admin), at [9]

[317] *Nursing and Midwifery Council (Practice Committees) (Constitution) Rules 2008*, SI 2008/3148, rule 6(11)

78 Absent Legal Assessor

78.1 The panel is not properly constituted in the absence of a legal assessor and may not proceed. A legal assessor must also be present during preliminary meetings.[318] If the legal assessor becomes unavailable during a hearing, proceedings must be adjourned until legal advice can be provided.

78.2 Substitution of a legal assessor is common and permissible, provided that the panel does not proceed at any stage in the assessor's absence and that the substitution is disclosed to the parties. In practice, it is frequently the case that the NMC is unable to secure a single legal assessor for the entire duration of a multi-day hearing. The present cadre of legal assessors can be safely relied upon to ensure continuity.

79 Absent Registrant's Representative

79.1 The absence of the registrant's representative does not of itself preclude continuation of proceedings. However, where a representative is unexpectedly unavailable, the panel must consider whether proceeding would be fair in the circumstances. Invariably, to proceed would be contrary to the interests of justice unless the registrant wished to proceed.

80 Order of Witnesses and Evidence

80.1 The panel's power to regulate the admission and management of evidence,[319] affords a broad discretion on panels in terms of case management. Panels are expected to take an active role in discharging their function and ensuring "that the case is

---

[318] FTP rule 18(2)(b)

[319] FTP rule 31

properly presented and that the relevant evidence is placed before it."[320]

80.2 The order in which witnesses are heard is classically a question of case management, hence panels enjoy broad discretion constrained by fairness to both parties and deference to the overarching objective.

80.3 Applications to hear witnesses out of turn, or to recall witnesses are therefore considered applications for case management directions.

81 Evidence in Rebuttal

81.1 Rebuttal evidence is not expressly defined in the FTP rules but is broadly admissible subject to permission of the panel applying a fairness and relevance test.[321]

82 Directing further inquiry

82.1 FTP proceedings are not conducted on a strictly adversarial model. Where it becomes apparent during a hearing that the evidential picture before the panel is incomplete, the panel is not confined to determining the case on the basis of the material presented. In appropriate circumstances, it may direct the regulator to undertake further inquiry or obtain additional evidence in order to enable the panel to make a fair and fully informed decision that properly protects the public.[322]

[320] *R (Council for the Regulation of Healthcare Professionals) v General Medical Council and Ruscillo* [2004] EWCA Civ 1356, at [80]

[321] FTP rule 31(1)

[322] FTP rule 22(5)

82.2 The panel should not regard itself as bound to find an allegation not proved merely because relevant evidence has not been adduced, where that evidence is clearly available and material to an issue it must decide; the panel must ensure "that the case is properly presented and that the relevant evidence is placed before it."[323]

82.3 In deciding whether to direct further inquiry, the panel should exercise judgement and restraint. Relevant considerations include whether the missing evidence is important to an issue the panel must (or should, if amendment is envisaged) determine; whether that evidence needs to be tested through witness examination; whether the panel can properly discharge its function without it; and whether directing further inquiry is consistent with the overarching objective of public protection. The panel must also consider the overall fairness of the proceedings, including fairness to the registrant, to witnesses, and to the regulator in the discharge of its statutory role, as well as the public interest in the expeditious disposal of the case.

83 Amendment of Charges

83.1 Panels may amend the charge or the facts on which it is based, at any stage before findings of fact are made, unless the amendment cannot be made "without injustice". [324] Before making any amendment, the panel must consider representations from the parties.[325]

83.2 In assessing whether an amendment can be made without injustice, the panel must consider the nature and scope of the

---

[323] *R (Council for the Regulation of Healthcare Professionals) v General Medical Council and Ruscillo* [2004] EWCA Civ 1356, at [80]

[324] FTP rule 28

[325] FTP rule 28(2)

proposed amendment, the reasons for it, the stage reached in the proceedings, along with any prejudice to the registrant. The closer an amendment is proposed to factual determination stage, the more exacting the scrutiny required. The availability of an adjournment does not of itself cure unfairness.

83.3 Amendments which introduce new factual allegations or materially alter the character of the case require particular caution, especially where they risk allowing the regulator to remedy deficiencies in its case at a late stage, or reflect new concerns which ought properly to have been through the case to answer process. Though there is no bar to including new concerns which have arisen since the initial case to answer decision,[326] the risk of injustice is increased where time to prepare a defence or seek identifiable disclosure is curtailed.

83.4 Within the assessment of fairness and injustice, however, panels must consider the public interest: "A professional disciplinary committee is entitled to make necessary amendments to the allegations before it, so as to avoid "undercharging"."[327] So too, the panel "should play a more proactive role than a judge presiding over a criminal trial in making sure that the case is properly presented and that the relevant evidence is placed before it."[328]

83.5 So too, may amendments serve in the registrant's favour. Amendments to clarify allegations, narrow or more accurately define their scope are likely to be considered fair, as allegations

---

326 *Rudling, R (On the Application of) v General Medical Council* [2018] EWHC 3582 (Admin), at [45]

327 *Professional Standards Authority v Health And Care Professions Council & Doree* [2017] EWCA Civ 319, at [54]

328 *R (Council for the Regulation of Healthcare Professionals) v General Medical Council and Ruscillo* [2004] EWCA Civ 1356, at [80]

"should be clearly particularised so that the person against whom it is made knows how the allegation is put."[329] Panels should take a proactive approach and may suggest amendment of their own volition, particularly where allegations are "hopelessly inadequately particularised."[330]

83.6 Panels must give clear reasons for allowing or refusing amendment, expressly addressing the test of fairness and injustice. Failure to do so may amount to procedural error.

84 Offering no evidence

84.1 In *Professional Standards Authority v Nursing and Midwifery Council & X*,[331] the High Court endorsed the position that "even though this is not expressly provided for in the Rules, it must be open to the NMC, in an appropriate case, to offer no evidence"[332] though "the cases in which it would be appropriate to offer no evidence will be rare."[333]

84.2 Where the NMC proposes to offer no evidence, "it is especially important, if the NMC considers that it is appropriate to offer no evidence, that it fully opens the case, so that the Committee is able to make a decision, informed by a sufficient knowledge of the facts, whether it is appropriate for the NMC to offer no

---

329 *Fish v General Medical Council* [2012] EWHC 1269 (Admin), at [69]

330 *Squier, R (On the Application of) v General Medical Council* [2015] EWHC 299 (Admin), at [55]

331 [2018] EWHC 70 (Admin)

332 *ibid*, at [55]

333 *ibid*, at [55]

evidence, or whether it should require the NMC to reconsider that view, and try and obtain more evidence."[334]

84.3 Where, prior to or at a substantive hearing, the regulator concludes that it is no longer in the public interest to pursue all or part of a charge, it may apply to a Fitness to Practise Committee to offer no evidence. This is not a unilateral withdrawal. The power rests with the panel, which must decide whether to approve the application. The regulator will ordinarily apply to offer no evidence only in limited circumstances, including where a particular part of the charge adds nothing to the overall seriousness of the case, where there is no longer a realistic prospect of proving some or all of the factual allegations, or where there is no longer a realistic prospect of a finding of current impairment.

84.4 Where an application to offer no evidence is made at a hearing, it must be raised at the outset, before pleas are taken. The panel will not invite the registrant to respond to the relevant charge or particulars until it has determined the application. The regulator must explain the background to the case, the steps taken in the investigation, and the reasons why it no longer seeks to proceed. The panel must be given sufficient information to understand both the seriousness of the original allegations and why continuation is no longer justified. The registrant must be given the opportunity to make representations, and the panel must receive legal advice before reaching its decision.

84.5 If the panel approves an application to offer no evidence on the whole of the charge, it must determine that the allegation is not well founded and give reasons, bringing the case (on the relevant allegation/s) to an end. If the application relates only

334 *ibid*, at [57]

to part of the charge, the panel may approve the application and amend the charge accordingly,[335] removing the relevant particulars so that the registrant is no longer required to answer them. In all cases, the panel must give clear reasons for its decision.

84.6 If the panel is not satisfied that the application should be granted, it may still call evidence of its own motion or direct further investigation,[336] which may require adjournment.

85 **Abuse of Process**

85.1 The FTP rules do not contain an express provision labelled "abuse of process". Panels retain power, however, to prevent proceedings from continuing where to do so would be unfair or would undermine the integrity of the regulatory process.

85.2 The scope of the doctrine is well established. In *R v Maxwell*,[337] Lord Dyson explained that proceedings may be stayed in two categories of case:

> (i) where it will be impossible to give the accused a fair trial; and (ii) where it offends the tribunal's sense of justice and propriety to be asked to try the case in the particular circumstances. In the first category, if a fair hearing cannot be achieved, no balancing exercise arises.[338]

85.3 The jurisdiction is to be exercised sparingly; to stay a case for abuse of process is "a rare step only to be taken in exceptional

[335] FTP rule 28

[336] FTP rule 22(5)

[337] [2010] UKSC 48

[338] *Maxwell*, at [13]

cases"[339], notwithstanding the strong public interest that serious allegations against professionals should ordinarily be heard and determined.

85.4 Abuse of process has been described as "something so unfair and wrong that the court should not allow a prosecutor to proceed with what is in all other respects a regular proceeding."[340] The focus is not on criticism of individual procedural decisions in isolation, but on whether the proceedings, viewed cumulatively, are or have become oppressive or incapable of delivering a fair hearing.

85.5 Many procedural difficulties can be cured by remedies short of stay, including adjournment, refusal or limitation of amendments, exclusion or restriction of evidence, or directions requiring further investigation. A stay is justified only where such remedies cannot cure the prejudice.

<u>Delay</u>

85.6 Delay is the most common basis upon which abuse of process is alleged, but delay is not abusive *per se* and is (unfortunately) characteristic of the FTP process. The relevant period by which delay is assessed is the time between the NMC receiving a complaint, and the hearing in question.[341]

> "The threshold of proving a breach of the reasonable time requirement is a high one, not easily crossed. But if the period which has elapsed is one which, on its face and without more, gives ground for real concern, two

339 *Haikel v General Medical Council* [2002] UKPC 37, at [15]

340 *Hui Chi-Ming v R* [1992] 1 AC 34 (PC), at 57B

341 *Okeke v Nursing and Midwifery Council* [2013] EWHC 714 (Admin), at [28]

> consequences follow. First, it is necessary [...] to look into the detailed facts and circumstances of the particular case. [...] Secondly, it is necessary for the [regulator] to explain and justify any lapse of time which appears to be excessive."[342]

85.7 The critical question is whether the passage of time has caused "real concern" leading to incurable prejudice; delay is only abusive where it has caused identifiable and incurable unfairness. Submissions should specify the forensic consequence said to arise from the delay, such as lost evidence or unavailable witnesses, and explain why that prejudice cannot be cured by case management or the panel's assessment of weight. Generalised complaint about systemic delay adds little.

Exceeding jurisdiction

85.8 Registrants occasionally advance abuse of process arguments on the basis that the regulator has exceeded its jurisdiction, either because the investigation was conducted inconsistently with the regulator's own published policies or because the subject matter of the investigation strays beyond the regulator's proper statutory remit.

85.9 Departures from investigative policy may "bite on the Tribunal's jurisdiction only through an abuse of process application."[343] However, mere departure is insufficient. The same high bar for incurable prejudice applies.

85.10 A second category of abuse argument arises where registrants contend that the regulator has moved impermissibly into areas protected by the European Convention on Human Rights.

---

342 *Dyer v Watson* [2004] 1 AC 379, at [52]

343 *Khan v General Medical Council* [2023] EWHC 3189 (Admin), at [26]

These arguments likewise do not operate as automatic bars to jurisdiction. The question is not whether Convention rights are engaged, but whether any interference is justified within the statutory purposes of professional regulation and whether the proceedings, viewed as a whole, remain fair and proportionate. Where a registrant contends that the regulator has impermissibly strayed into protected territory, that contention must again be articulated through an abuse of process application focused on unfairness, not as a challenge to jurisdiction *per se*.

Article 6 ECHR

85.11 Where a panel concludes that procedural developments have rendered a fair hearing impossible, the case falls within the first *Maxwell* category and must be stayed. In such circumstances the panel must not engage in a balancing exercise between fairness to the registrant and inconvenience to the regulator, witnesses, or the public interest in expedition.

Article 8 ECHR

85.12 Article 8 protects private and family life, including reputation. "It has, however, always been recognised that misconduct may qualify even though committed in the professional's private life, so long as it has a sufficient impact on his professional reputation or that of the profession as a whole."[344] For example, "requirements to act with integrity and to act so as to maintain public trust [...] are requirements which will, on occasions require the [...] the Tribunal to adjudicate on a professional

[344] *Gleeson v Social Work England* [2024] EWHC 3 (Admin), at [101]

person's private life. Common sense dictates that such cases must and will arise."[345]

85.13 The question to be applied is whether the interference is proportionate; a question to be considered anxiously:

> There can be no hard and fast rule either that regulation [...] may never be directed to the regulated person's private life, or that any/every aspect of her private life is liable to scrutiny. But [...rules...] may reach into private life only when conduct that is part of a person's private life realistically touches on her practise of the profession [...] or the standing of the profession [...] Any such conduct must be qualitatively relevant. It must, in a way that is demonstrably relevant, engage one or other of the standards of behaviour which are set out in or necessarily implicit from the [rules]. In this way, the required fair balance is properly struck between the right to respect to private life and the public interest in the regulation of the [...] profession. Regulators will do well to recognise that it is all too easy to be dogmatic without knowing it; popular outcry is not proof that a particular set of events gives rise to any matter falling within a regulator's remit.[346]

85.14 In practical terms, Article 8 arguments are more often deployed with greater force at the stage of determining misconduct than as a basis for abuse of process. Where the conduct relied upon lies within a registrant's private life, the critical question is whether there is a sufficient professional nexus to justify regulatory intervention in those circumstances.

---

[345] *Beckwith v Solicitors Regulation Authority* [2020] EWHC 3231, at [50]

[346] *Beckwith*, at [54]

Article 10 ECHR

85.15 Article 10 issues arise where allegations concern speech, expression, or public commentary, including social media. The courts have repeatedly confirmed that professional regulation may extend beyond the workplace; that "professional discipline, rightly, sits relatively lightly on its members outside the workplace, but it is never entirely absent where conduct in public is concerned."[347]

85.16 Challenges to broadly framed professional standards on Article 10 grounds have been consistently rejected, with the courts accepting that "any attempt to provide absolute precision would be undesirable given the context, which is regulation of a profession in the public interest. One cannot legislate for all circumstances in advance. There needs to be sufficient flexibility so as to protect the public interest as new factual situations arise."[348]

85.17 The maintenance of public confidence in the profession, part of the NMC's overarching objective,[349] is a "legitimate aim" to warrant interference with Article 10 rights such that a rule requiring registrants not to bring the profession into disrepute "corresponds to a pressing social need and, making all due allowance for the wide parameters of the Article 10(1) right".[350]

85.18 In abuse of process terms, Article 10 rarely mandates a stay. Its relevance lies in cases where procedural developments, such as

[347] *Ngole v University of Sheffield (HCPC intervening)* [2017] EWHC 2669 (Admin), at [175]

[348] *R (Pitt and Tyas) v General Pharmaceutical Council* [2017] EWHC 809 (Admin), at [47]

[349] Article 3(4A)(b)

[350] *Khan v Bar Standards Board* [2018] EWHC 2184 (Admin), at [65]

late amendment or re-characterisation, transform proceedings into a materially different speech-based case without adequate notice or opportunity to respond, thereby compounding.

Article 9 ECHR

85.19 Article 9 protects freedom of thought, conscience and religion, including the manifestation of belief, but does not place belief-based conduct beyond regulatory scrutiny. Article 9 authorities on conscientious objection confirm that objectives such as maintaining public trust may constitute legitimate aims justifying interference.[351]

85.20 Gender-critical and religious beliefs are protected under Article 9.[352] However, Article 9 is a qualified right; professional standards restricting manifestation may be proportionate where they pursue sufficiently important objectives, are rationally connected, and strike a fair balance.[353]

85.21 As with Article 10, Article 9 interference is unlikely to provide a free-standing basis for a stay. Its relevance lies more easily in cases where panels are asked to consider whether belief-based conduct may amount to misconduct.

86 Pleas in bar

86.1 Plea in bar may arise where a registrant contends that regulatory proceedings are precluded because the matter has already been determined. In professional discipline, these arguments most

---

351 *Ngole v University of Sheffield* [2017] EWHC 2669 (Admin), at [100]

352 *Sutcliffe v Secretary of State for Education* [2024] EWHC 1878 (Admin), at [55.1]

353 *Sutcliffe*, at [60]

take the form of *res judicata*, cause of action estoppel, or the closely related concept of *autrefois*.

Previous regulator action

86.2 In "case where there have been two successive sets of disciplinary proceedings"[354] by the same regulator on the same facts, there is is no principled reason why doctrines of finality should not apply: "the principles of cause of action estoppel should [...] apply to proceedings before a disciplinary tribunal."[355] Professional discipline is not immune from the application of *res judicata*.

86.3 Although the language of *autrefois acquit* and *autrefois convict* is sometimes used by analogy, "it is not the principles of autrefois convict which apply to disciplinary proceedings, which are civil in nature."[356]

86.4 The practical consequence is that pleas in bar in professional discipline are properly analysed through the lens of *res judicata* and cause of action estoppel, rather than through a direct transplantation of criminal law doctrines. Where a regulator seeks to bring successive proceedings arising from the same factual matrix, the tribunal must consider whether the later proceedings impermissibly seek to relitigate matters that could and should have been advanced in the earlier case. If so, fairness and finality may require the proceedings to be barred.

86.5 However, *Coke-Wallis* does not establish a general prohibition on further regulatory action in all circumstances. The

---

[354] *R (on the application of Coke-Wallis) v Institute of Chartered Accountants in England and Wales* [2011] UKSC 1, at [25]

[355] *Coke-Wallis*, at [29]

[356] *Coke-Wallis*, at [59]

applicability of a plea in bar depends on careful analysis of what was previously determined, the scope of the earlier proceedings, and whether the later case truly involves the same cause of action.

Action by other bodies

86.6 Pleas in bar operate narrowly. They may prevent successive proceedings by the same regulator where a matter has already been finally determined. They do not, without more, prevent a regulator from exercising its own statutory jurisdiction in respect of conduct which has been adjudged by another regulator or body. The fact that the conduct of a registrant might fall within the regulatory remit of another professional body does not, of itself, preclude NMC proceedings:[357]

> The fact that there may be an overlap with another statutory regulatory regime (here the SRA) does not, in my judgement, oust the jurisdiction of the Defendant in this regard. Membership of each profession brings separate regulatory oversight; each regulator has the untrammelled jurisdiction to investigate its own registrants and the Defendant cannot delegate its functions [...] to the SRA. It will no doubt be unusual, but that may mean that an individual with dual registration could face separate investigation by two different regulators over substantially the same matter.[358]

86.7 Similarly, the NMC is not estopped from proceeding against a registrant where the Crown Prosecution Service decides not to

[357] *Ogunsanya & Anor v General Medical Council* [2020] EWHC 1500 (QB), at [38]

[358] *Ogunsanya*, at [39]

prosecute.[359] Nor is the regulator necessarily prevented from continuing FTP proceedings where a registrant has been acquitted by a criminal court of an offence:

> professional conduct panels do not require the criminal standard of proof but apply the civil standard. [..] It is important to bear in mind that the purpose of criminal proceedings is the imposition of a sanction for breach of the criminal law; regulators have no choice whether or not a prosecution is mounted (usually by the CPS) [...] The focus of regulators is to maintain the standards and integrity of the profession to ensure that public confidence is and can be maintained and it would not be in the public interest for a form of regulatory arbitrage to take place if there was an 'either/or' approach to whether proceedings should be pursued through the criminal courts or by the regulator. [...] The test must not be whether a second bite of the cherry might secure a 'better' outcome but, rather, what is in the public interest, viewing the case through the lens of the obligations placed on the regulator. [...] It is therefore important to confirm that although it is not inherently unfair to bring misconduct charges against a professional who has already been acquitted in the criminal courts, this does not mean that there will not be circumstances in which it may well be unfair to proceed. [...] Regulators must each determine how they go about achieving their regulatory objectives and, bearing those objectives in mind, faithfully apply the well-known principles engaged within the concept of abuse of process."[360]

---

[359] *Khan v General Medical Council* [2023] EWHC 3189 (Admin), at [32]

[360] *Ashraf v General Dental Council* [2014] EWHC 2618 (Admin), at [33] – [36]

86.8 Practitioners must therefore be alert to the frequently-encountered scenario of the same incident (often, an assault), culminating in a not guilty verdict before a criminal court, yet being found proved to the civil standard in FTP proceedings.

87 Bias

87.1 Bias is conceptually distinct from abuse of process. Abuse of process asks whether proceedings have become so unfair that they cannot properly continue. Bias asks whether the decision-maker is, or appears to be, incapable of approaching the case with the requisite impartiality. Where apparent bias is established, the integrity of the adjudicative process is compromised and the decision will ordinarily be vitiated.

87.2 Allegations of bias should be advanced without personal criticism of individual decision-makers. The focus is institutional and constitutional: "justice should not only be done, but should manifestly and undoubtedly be seen to be done."[361] A recusal decision is neither an admission nor a finding of wrongdoing. It is a mechanism for protecting public confidence and ensuring that the process is fair.

87.3 The *Porter v Magill*[362] test applies, namely whether the fair-minded and informed observer, having considered the facts, would conclude that there is a real possibility that the tribunal is biased. The test is not whether there is or has been bias, nor does a decision to recuse suggest or concede the same. No finding of bias is necessary. The question is solely whether there

---

[361] *R v Sussex Justices, ex p McCarthy* [1924] 1 KB 256, at 259

[362] [2002] 2 AC 357

is a real possibility.[363] If "there is real ground for doubt, that doubt should be resolved in favour of recusal."[364]

87.4 That a panel member shares a profession with the registrant "will of itself come nowhere near establishing an appearance of bias."[365] However, where a panel member holds an appointment outside of their NMC engagement of particular proximity to the registrant or any witness, an appearance of bias may arise.[366] When considering whether the circumstances lead a fair-minded and informed observer to conclude that there is a real possibility that the tribunal was biased "it is important not to draw "fine distinctions". What matters is the impression that would be left on the fair-minded and informed observer."[367]

87.5 Where the issue of bias and recusal arises after a hearing has commenced, rather than at its outset, the remedy sought should be recusal of the panel *in toto*:

> "A panel which has sat for ten days (as the Committee has here) will be bound to have discussed the case in detail. It is impossible to know how influential the views of the individual panel members have been. If one member is tainted by apparent bias, the Committee's decision will be vitiated."[368]

---

363 *Nwabueze v General Medical Council* [2000] UKPC 16, at [21]

364 *Locabail (UK) Ltd v Bayfield Properties Ltd & Anor* [1999] EWCA Civ 3004, at [25]

365 *Kimmance v General Medical Council* [2016] EWHC 1808 (Admin), at [22]

366 See: *Suleman v General Optical Council* [2023] EWHC 2110 (Admin)

367 *Suleman*, at [29]

368 *Suleman*, at [32]

CHAPTER NINE

COMMON EVIDENTIAL DISPUTES

88 Admissibility generally

88.1 FTP proceedings are not governed by the strict rules of evidence applicable in other courts or tribunals. Admissibility is regulated by FTP rule 31(1), which confers a broad discretion on the panel to admit evidence (of any sort) whether or not such evidence would be admissible in civil proceedings, subject only to relevance and fairness and having taken the advice of the legal assessor.

88.2 Relevance and fairness must both be made out before admission. Evidence may be factually connected to the background of a case yet inadmissible because it does not assist the panel in determining the issues it must decide, or because its admission would compromise the fairness of the proceedings.

88.3 Admissibility issues commonly arise at the bundle stage, where draft bundles include a wide range of investigative material such as employer documents, internal reviews, supervision records, and correspondence. Practitioners should scrutinise such material in advance and identify content that is irrelevant or unfair. Where redactions are agreed, the issue can be resolved on the papers. Where agreement cannot be reached, admissibility should be determined by way of a preliminary application.

88.4 Applications to adduce or exclude evidence should be framed explicitly as applications under rule 31. The rule provides the sole procedural gateway for admissibility.

88.5 Panels should rule expressly on such applications, identifying whether material is admitted or excluded under FTP rule 31 and on what basis. It is not uncommon for parts of documents to be admitted with irrelevant or unfair passages redacted. Where admissibility is challenged at a final hearing, the panel will consider the evidence *de bene esse*, putting out of its mind any material subsequently ruled inadmissible; "the mere fact that [contested] pages [are] contained in the bundle, as opposed to being kept separate until after the determination of the admissibility point, does not amount to a procedural error or give rise to a decision that was wrong."[369]

89 **Hearsay**

89.1 Hearsay evidence is a recurrent feature of fitness to practise proceedings and should be approached as a structural reality of the regulatory process. Panels are not bound by the strict rules of admissibility applicable in criminal courts. The governing test is whether the evidence is fair and relevant. That discretion is wide but not unconfined, and practitioners should be prepared to challenge both the admission of hearsay and the weight ultimately attached to it.

89.2 Despite the frequency with which hearsay is relied upon in FTP proceedings, admission of hearsay "should not be regarded as a routine matter."[370] The starting point is "the critical distinction

[369] *Mansaray v Nursing and Midwifery Council* [2023] EWHC 730 (Admin), at [65]

[370] *Thorneycroft v Nursing and Midwifery Council* [2014] EWHC 1565 (Admin), at [45(1.1)]

between admissibility and weight [...] as a matter of law, [the panel] must first determine admissibility as a question of fairness before considering the question of weight."[371]

89.3 When considering whether it is fair to admit hearsay, the panel will consider that there is "no absolute rule whether under Article 6 or in common law entitling a person facing disciplinary proceedings to cross-examine witnesses on whose evidence the allegations against him are based. Nor does such an entitlement arise automatically by reason of the fact that the evidence of the witness in question is the sole or decisive basis of the evidence against him."[372] Admissibility depends on the facts of the case. In particular, the panel should have regard to: the existence or otherwise of a good and cogent reason for the non-attendance;[373] the nature and extent of the challenge to the content of the hearsay evidence;[374] whether there was any suggestion that the witnesses had reasons to fabricate their allegations;[375] whether the applicant party has taken reasonable steps to secure the attendance of the witness;[376] and whether the registrant had prior notice that the evidence was to be relied upon as hearsay.[377]

---

371 *El Karout v Nursing and Midwifery Council* [2019] EWHC 28 (Admin), at [128]

372 *Bonhoeffer, R (On the Application Of) v General Medical Council* [2011] EWHC 1585 (Admin), at [39]

373 *Thorneycroft*, at [45(1.3)]

374 *Thorneycroft*, at [56(ii)]

375 *Thorneycroft*, at [56(iii)]

376 *Thorneycroft*, at [56(vi)]

377 *Thorneycroft*, at [56(vii)]

89.4 Consideration of the other evidence to be called is particularly important. Where hearsay evidence is the sole or decisive evidence in relation to the charges, the decision whether or not to admit requires that the panel "must be satisfied that the evidence is demonstrably reliable, or alternatively that there is some means of testing its reliability.[378] "In order to assess the degree of demonstrable reliability and the capability of it being tested in order to decide whether to admit it, it is to some extent necessary to weigh the evidence itself."[379]

89.5 In considering what other evidence exists, and the nature and extent of challenge to the content of hearsay evidence, the panel may consider any statement previously provided by the registrant or any admissions. "In order to evaluate whether admitting the hearsay would meet the 'fair and relevant' test it [is] important for the preliminary tribunal to know what the issues in the case [are]."[380] This does not shift the burden of proof, which remains on the regulator, but admissibility is assessed by reference to the case actually being tried, not a hypothetical one.

89.6 Submissions on a hearsay application should be structured as an FTP rule 31 fairness analysis, identifying the precise evidential item and the factual issue it is said to prove. The core of the submission should then separate admissibility from weight and address, in order, the features which bear on fairness: why the witness is absent and what steps have been taken to secure attendance (including a detailed chronology of attempts and correspondence); whether the registrant had proper notice; and

---

[378] *Thorneycroft*, at [45]; *El Karout*, at [101]

[379] *Mansaray v Nursing and Midwifery Council* [2023] EWHC 730 (Admin), at [56]

[380] *Lee v General Medical Council* [2025] EWHC 3347 (Admin), at [30]

the extent to which the hearsay is disputed in substance. An important exercise is to identify where the hearsay sits within the overall evidential matrix; whether it is sole or decisive on any matters the panel has to determine. If so, submissions should articulate either the counterbalancing measures relied upon by the party seeking admission (corroboration, contemporaneous documents, internal consistency, prior accounts, admissions, or other mechanisms by which reliability can be tested such as asking questions of other witnesses), or the specific forensic prejudice relied upon by the party seeking exclusion (for example, the inability to test credibility on a determinative issue, or the absence of any meaningful substitute for cross-examination).

89.7 Where hearsay is admitted, the panel must continue to treat such evidence with caution when making findings of fact. The absence of cross-examination, the timing of the statement, the possibility of honest mistake, and any motive to complain must feature in the reasoning as to the weight which might safely be apportioned. Reference is frequently made in legal advice to panels to the helpful (though not binding) considerations in s.4, Civil Evidence Act 1995.

90 Character evidence

Good character

90.1 Evidence of good character is relevant in FTP proceedings,[381] but only in limited respects.

90.2 "It is now clearly established that, just as in a criminal trial, in professional disciplinary proceedings good character is relevant

[381] Therefore meeting one of the admissibility criteria under FTP rule 31.

to both credibility and propensity;"[382] that is "how reasonable it is to believe or disbelieve what an individual says [and] the probability that they have misconducted themselves."[383] However, evidence of good character "cannot afford a defence in itself." [384]

90.3 The weight to be attached to good character evidence is "in the last resort a matter for the Tribunal"[385] considering the relevance of the good character and other evidence available.

90.4 Understandably, "the weight given to an unblemished record may properly be less in the case of a [registrant] at an early stage in her career than a [registrant] with an established track record."[386]

90.5 Though it is preferable that a panel "set out its understanding of the legal position, namely that good character evidence is relevant to the issues of both propensity and credibility […] it is not a legal requirement."[387] Authority "does not support the proposition that it is a misdirection in law not to give a good character direction"[388] during legal advice to the panel; panels are "an expert, professional jury which does not need the sort of 'good character direction' one sees in criminal trials […] and

---

[382] *Khan v General Medical Council* [2021] EWHC 374 (Admin), at [86]

[383] *Sawati v General Medical Council* [2022] EWHC 283 (Admin), at [54]; *Wisson v Health Professions Council* [2013] EWHC 1036 (Admin), at [41]–[44]

[384] *Donkin v Law Society* [2007] EWHC 414 (Admin), at [25]

[385] *Donkin*, at [25]

[386] *Sawati v General Medical Council* [2022] EWHC 283 (Admin), at [69]

[387] *Nwosu v Solicitors Regulation Authority* [2023] EWHC 2405 (KB), at [45]

[388] *Vitalis v Nursing And Midwifery Council* [2017] EWHC 3281 (Admin), at [21]

does not need to have demonstrated that it took the [registrant's] good character into account by express reference to these trite principles in the body of its Judgment."[389] However, error arises where relevant good character evidence does not "play any part" in the tribunal's evaluation of issues such as dishonesty.[390]

90.6 Further, a panel is entitled to proceed on the basis that a registrant or witness is of good character unless evidence to the contrary is adduced: "all witnesses are of good character unless the Panel hears to the contrary," [391] particularly as "all or nearly all registrants in professions such as nursing, where higher standards of integrity are required, are likely to be persons of good character. It will therefore, in many cases, be superfluous to repeat that trite proposition in a particular case."[392]

90.7 At the sanction stage, good character may be relied on in mitigation. Prior good character is of limited assistance, however, given the overarching objective. "Because orders made by the Tribunal are not primarily punitive, it follows that considerations which would ordinarily weigh in mitigation of punishment have less effect on the exercise of this jurisdiction than on the ordinary run of sentences imposed in criminal cases [...] The reputation of the profession is more important than the fortunes of any individual member. Membership of a profession brings many benefits, but that is a part of the price."[393] The need to uphold the overarching objective "is constant, regardless of the nature of the gross misconduct under

---

[389] *Shaw & Anor v Logue* [2014] EWHC 5 (Admin), at [182]

[390] *Donkin*, at [25]

[391] *Gopakumar v General Medical Council* [2008] EWCA Civ 309, at [34]

[392] *Vitalis,* at [21]

[393] *Bolton v Law Society* [1994] 1 W.L.R. 512, at 519B-E

consideration. What may vary will be the extent to which the particular gross misconduct threatens the preservation of such confidence and respect. The more it does so, the less weight can be given to personal mitigation."[394]

Bad character

90.8 Evidence of bad character is admissible through the relevance and fairness gateway of FTP rule 31.

90.9 The admission of bad character evidence against a registrant at the facts stage is atypical. Such evidence (typically prior disciplinary outcomes or investigations) may, exceptionally, be relevant to "the particular circumstances of the case"[395] in which the alleged misconduct occurred and by which it should be judged, particularly where the alleged misconduct involved breach of a prior order.

90.10 Whether relating to the registrant or a witness, "convictions for [...] offences of dishonesty or convictions for any offence following a plea of not guilty, where the person concerned gave evidence that was disbelieved or for that matter evidence that a person's evidence was disbelieved in a civil case, is material that is at least potentially relevant to an assessment of credibility."[396]

90.11 Prior findings and regulatory history are plainly relevant at the impairment and sanction stages, where the panel is required to assess current risk, insight, remediation, and the protection of the public. At that stage, the FTP rules envisage the panel being

[394] *Williams, R (On the Application of) v Police Appeals Tribunal* [2016] EWHC 2708 (Admin), at [66]

[395] *Roylance v General Medical Council* [1999] UKPC 16, at [38]

[396] *H, R (On the Application of) v Nursing and Midwifery Council* [2013] EWHC 4258 (Admin), at [18]

made aware of relevant previous determinations.[397] Panels must avoid double counting and ensure that adverse history is used to inform proportionality and risk, not to punish the registrant again for past misconduct, though prior disciplinary history may properly be treated as an aggravating feature.

91 Investigation outcomes

91.1 Too often, panels become privy to material arising from internal disciplinary processes, employer investigations, safeguarding enquiries, or other supervisory or managerial fact-finding exercises which disclose the decisions of local or earlier investigations. This may include investigation reports, disciplinary outcomes, grievance determinations, or letters recording internal decisions. Such material is commonly referred to, as shorthand, as "*Enemuwe* material".

91.2 The legal position is clear. Evidence of the findings or outcomes of internal investigations is inadmissible. Panels must determine the facts for themselves on the admissible evidence properly before them. They are not entitled to rely upon, or be influenced by, conclusions reached by others operating under different procedures, standards, and purposes. The principle is articulated in emphatic terms in *Enemuwe v Nursing and Midwifery Council*:[398]

> What [the panel] should in fact have done was decline to admit any evidence by any means of the outcome of the supervisory investigation, and they should have treated the findings and decision of [that investigation] as

[397] FTP rule 24(13)(c)

[398] [2015] EWHC 2081 (Admin) , at [83]

completely irrelevant and excluded from their consideration by operation of rule 31(1).

91.3 The rationale is straightforward. Internal investigations are conducted for different purposes, under different legal frameworks, and frequently without the procedural safeguards required in FTP proceedings. They may involve limited disclosure, no oral evidence, no cross-examination, and standards driven by employment policy rather than statutory regulation. To permit their findings to influence a panel risks substituting managerial conclusions for the panel's own independent fact-finding function.

91.4 In practical terms, *Enemuwe* material should be redacted from hearing bundles. Where it appears within witness statements, reports, or exhibits, practitioners should seek its removal in advance. If such material persists into the final bundle, or emerges in oral evidence despite redaction, it is important that the panel is expressly directed to disregard it. Submissions should make clear that the panel must exclude the material from its consideration entirely when determining facts.

91.5 A variant to the *Enemuwe* rule applies to the factual findings of civil courts, which may be treated as *prima facie* proof of matters alleged. However, the registrant must be permitted to challenge the correctness of the conclusion and to call evidence if desired.[399] The same applies to coronial verdicts and narrative findings.[400]

---

[399] *General Medical Council v Spackman* [1943] AC 628

[400] *Towuaghantse v General Medical Council (Rev 2)* [2021] EWHC 681 (Admin), at [35]

92 Expert and opinion evidence

92.1 As a general principle, witnesses may give evidence of fact but not opinion. The panel must reach its own conclusions on the issues it is required to determine, rather than deferring to the views of others. Opinion evidence risks usurping that function unless it falls within a recognised exception and will never be admissible in respect of the questions of misconduct and impairment, which are the preserve of the panel.

92.2 There are two well-established exceptions to the general prohibition. First, expert witnesses may give opinion evidence on matters requiring specialist knowledge outside the experience of the tribunal, provided the opinion is confined to that field of expertise.[401] The FTP rules envisage the use of independent expert evidence in that traditional sense.[402] Second, non-expert witnesses may express opinions that are incidental to their factual evidence and within ordinary lay competence, such as estimates of speed or distance. In professional discipline contexts, this second category has seen expansion.

Independent experts

92.3 The first category of expert evidence in FTP proceedings is not bound strictly by the Criminal Procedure Rules or CPR Part 35, but in practice such reports carry the same declarations. The panel remains the sole decision-maker on facts, misconduct, impairment and sanction. Expert evidence exists to assist the panel, not to determine those questions for it.

---

401 *R v Turner* [1975] QB 834, 841F – 842B

402 FTP rule 18(5)(e)

92.4 A panel is not bound to accept expert evidence even where uncontested,[403] but where a panel rejects the evidence of an expert witness, it must explain why it has done so.

92.5 Where competing expert evidence is called by either side, the panel should endeavour in its reasons to "provide an explanation as to why he has accepted the evidence of one expert and rejected that of another."[404] Reasons shall be deficient where they are such that the parties "do not know what, if any, view the committee formed about the difference of opinion."[405]

<u>Factual witnesses</u>

92.6 Such is the nature of FTP proceedings that witnesses of fact frequently possess professional or technical expertise; many are regulated professionals working in areas of particular specialism. Panels should not assume that opinion evidence is admissible only if given by an independent expert formally instructed for the purposes of the proceedings. The principles of Part 35 governing instructed expert evidence "only regulate the use of a particular category of expert evidence"[406] and do not preclude the admission of other expert or quasi-expert opinion where it is otherwise admissible.

92.7 A registrant may give evidence as to why consider that their conduct did not fall below the standard of care reasonably expected and to do so by reference to their knowledge and expertise in the particular field. That such evidence may lack

[403] *Tui UK Ltd v Griffiths* [2023] UKSC 48, at [61] – [70]

[404] *English v Emery Reimbold & Strick Limited* [2002] EWCA Civ 605, at [20]

[405] *Rimmer v General Dental Council* [2011] EWHC 3438 (Admin), at [17]

[406] *Hoyle v Rogers* [2014] EWCA Civ 257, at [63]

the objectivity of an independent expert goes to its cogency or weight, not its admissibility.[407]

92.8 So too, a witness with relevant specialist expertise "who is giving factual evidence may also proffer (a) statements of opinion which are reasonably related to the facts within his knowledge and (b) relevant comments based upon his own experience."[408] This category of opinion evidence is particularly common in FTP proceedings, particularly where witnesses are asked to give evidence on clinical decision making and local practice.

92.9 The panel should note in cases where no independent expert is available that non-expert opinion evidence does not carry the same status as expert evidence and must be evaluated with caution. Panels must satisfy themselves that the witness genuinely possesses the relevant expertise and that the opinion remains within it.

Registrant panel members

92.10 Given the presence of registrant panel members, it is not uncommon in FTP proceedings to encounter situations where evidence strays beyond "ordinary human experience"[409] and into matters of medical practice, which might otherwise be considered areas of expertise. Reliance by the panel on the expertise of the registrant member(s) is not inherently improper, but "the rules of natural justice preclude members of a specialist tribunal including expert members from giving evidence to themselves which the parties have no opportunity

[407] *DN v London Borough of Greenwich* [2004] EWCA Civ 1659, at [25] – [26]

[408] *Multiplex Constructions (UK) Ltd v Cleveland Bridge UK Ltd* (No. 6) [2008] EWHC 2220 (TCC), at [672]

[409] *R v Turner* [1975] QB 834, 841G

to challenge and that where a specialist tribunal drawing on its own knowledge and experience independently identifies an important fact or matter which may influence its decision but which has not been the subject of evidence adduced by or submissions advanced by the parties, it should state this openly and give the parties an opportunity to seek to adduce evidence and/or make submissions on it."[410]

---

[410] *Lawrence v General Medical Council* [2012] EWHC 464 (Admin), at [229]

CHAPTER TEN

REVIEWS

93 **Purpose**

93.1 Review hearings are frequently misunderstood. They are not an addendum to the substantive hearing, nor a tick-box exercise on the path to restoration or strike-off. They are a substantive jurisdiction in their own right, governed by the overarching statutory objective and requiring a different analytical approach to that applied at the original hearing.

93.2 The rationale for review hearings is protective; they exist because fitness to practise is not static. Risk may reduce, insight may develop, and circumstances may change. Review hearings allow the regulator to reassess whether ongoing restriction remains necessary to protect the public, maintain confidence in the profession, and uphold professional standards; they are a key mechanism by which the regulator ensures that its powers are exercised proportionately

94 **Orders subject to review**

94.1 Caution orders may be reviewed at the request of the registrant, or the NMC.[411]

94.2 Conditions of practice orders and suspension orders must be reviewed before they expire,[412] unless the issuing panel directed

---

[411] Article 30(2)

[412] Article 30(1)

that the order should lapse on expiry,[413] and may be reviewed at any other time at the request of the registrant or the NMC.[414]

94.3 Strike-off orders are final, subject only to appeal and to the separate jurisdiction relating to restoration.

94.4 Conditions of practice orders are intended to permit safe practice subject to defined restrictions, supervision, or requirements. Reviews assess whether those conditions have been complied with, whether they continue to address the identified risk, and whether they remain necessary.

94.5 Suspension order reviews are often pivotal moments, because escalation to strike-off may become available if impairment persists.

94.6 Orders imposed by consent are reviewed in the same way as contested orders; agreement does not dilute the panel's statutory duties.

95 The scope of a review hearing

95.1 Reviewing panels are bound by the original findings of fact. They cannot revisit whether allegations were proved, nor entertain arguments that the original decision was wrong. Challenges to the original decision lie by appeal; allowing a registrant to go behind the facts established would be "alien to the generally accepted conception of a review as a vehicle for monitoring the steps taken by the registrant towards securing professional rehabilitation."[415]

---

[413] Article 29(8A)

[414] Article 30(2)

[415] *Khan v General Pharmaceutical Council* [2016] UKSC 64, at [31]

95.2 The same constraint applies to panels; a panel may not extend or increase a sanction because it disagrees with the seriousness assessment made originally. "It can never be a proper ground for the exercise of the power to extend the period of suspension that the period originally directed was insufficient to reflect the gravity of the original offence or offences."[416]

95.3 Extension of an order may therefore only be based on the registrant's current fitness to practise (insight, remediation, risk, skills): what the panel must do is assess current impairment. In so doing, the panel will adopt the factual background and consider the registrant's conduct since the original hearing and any previous reviews.

96 **Process at a review hearing**

96.1 Review hearings are often heard by a differently constituted panel. There is no requirement for continuity. Panels rely heavily on the written determinations from the substantive hearing and prior reviews, which frame the case.

96.2 The structure of a review hearing is prescribed by FTP rule 25. The presenter opens by setting out the background, the order imposed, and any relevant evidence and previous determinations.[417] The registrant then bears the evidential burden of adducing material relied upon to demonstrate change.[418] The panel then deliberates and disposes of the case by reference to current impairment and proportionality, giving reasons. This procedural sequence reflects the limited and forward-looking nature of the review jurisdiction.

---

416 *Taylor v General Medical Council* [1990] 2 AC 539, at 545

417 FTP rule 25(2)(a)

418 FTP rule 25(2)(b)

97 Preparation for a review hearing

97.1 Effective preparation begins early. Review hearings are evidence-driven. Assertions of improvement or learning carry little weight without corroboration. Preparation involves identifying what has changed since the last hearing. This may include completion of courses, supervised practice, reflective work, compliance with conditions, health treatment, or changes in employment. The narrative should be forward-looking and structured around risk reduction.

97.2 Defensive or adversarial approaches are rarely effective. Panels expect realism, candour, and a clear understanding of the original concerns.

98 Evidence at review hearings

98.1 Registrant evidence is important but rarely sufficient on its own. Reflective statements should demonstrate understanding of the findings, acceptance of responsibility where appropriate, and learning. Generic expressions of remorse are unlikely to satisfy a panel. Independent evidence is often decisive. Employer and supervisor reports carry significant weight, particularly where they address the specific risks identified in the original decision. Reports should be detailed, balanced, and current.

98.2 Where impairment relates to insufficient knowledge of English, the NMC may direct that the registrant undertake an examination or assessment prior to the review hearing.[419]

---

[419] FTP rule 25A(2)(a)

98.3 Where impairment relates to health, up-to-date medical evidence is essential, together with evidence of engagement with treatment and insight into management of risk.

99 **Insight and remediation in practice**

99.1 Insight is paramount. Panels look for more than acknowledgment of outcome. Insight involves understanding why the conduct occurred, recognising its impact, and demonstrating how recurrence will be prevented.

99.2 In *Dhoorah v Nursing and Midwifery Council*,[420] the pertinent authorities were succinctly distilled thus:

> [21] Guidance on how to consider the question of impairment on review was set out in *Abraheam v General Medical Council*,[421] in which Blake J stated:
>
> > "23. ... the statutory context for the Rule relating to reviews must mean that the review has to consider whether all the concerns raised in the original finding of impairment through misconduct have been sufficiently addressed to the Panel's satisfaction. In practical terms there is a persuasive burden on the practitioner at a review to demonstrate that he or she has fully acknowledged why past professional performance was deficient and through insight, application, education, supervision or other achievement sufficiently addressed the past impairments."
>
> [21] In *Yusuff v General Medical Council* [2018] EWHC 13 (Admin), Yip J addressed the particular difficulty that

[420] [2020] EWHC 3356 (Admin)

[421] [2008] EWHC 183 (Admin)

can arise where (as here) a registrant maintains their innocence:

> "18. It would be wrong to equate maintenance of innocence with a lack of insight. However, continued denial of the misconduct found proved will be relevant to the Tribunal's considerations on review... refusal to accept the misconduct and failure to tell the truth during the hearing will be very relevant to the initial sanction. At the review stage, things will have moved on. The registrant may be able to demonstrate insight without accepting that the findings at the original hearing were true. The Sanctions Guidance makes it clear that at a review hearing the Tribunal is to consider whether the doctor has fully appreciated the gravity of the offence and must be satisfied that patients will not be put at risk if he resumes practice. A want of candour and continued dishonesty may be taken into account by the Tribunal in reaching its conclusions on impairment..."

99.3 Attendance at review hearings is therefore important. Non-attendance may be interpreted as disengagement, particularly where unexplained. Panels frequently test insight through questioning. Registrants should be prepared to answer candidly and specifically. Rehearsed or formulaic answers are often counterproductive.

99.4 Where difficulties have arisen, candour is generally more effective than minimisation. Panels respond better to openness coupled with a credible plan. Unworkable conditions should be raised proactively as partial compliance is rarely greeted with enthusiasm. Practitioners should propose realistic variations supported by evidence.

99.5 Remediation must be targeted. Panels expect a clear link between the original concerns and the steps taken to address them. Generic or unrelated courses are rarely persuasive.

99.6 Partial insight is common. Panels may acknowledge progress while concluding that impairment remains. Practitioners should address this honestly rather than overstating the position.

100 **Risk assessment at review**

100.1 Risk assessment is forward-looking. Panels assess the likelihood of repetition and the seriousness of potential harm. The absence of further incidents does not automatically resolve risk, and compliance with conditions is expected. Compliance alone does not justify revocation unless it demonstrates that underlying risk has been addressed rather than merely controlled.

101 **Outcomes**

101.1 The panel may revoke the order, vary or replace it, extend it, escalate to a more restrictive order, or impose no order. In practice, review outcomes turn on a small number of judgements: risk reduction, depth of insight, and necessity of restriction. A panel may not, however, impose an order which was not available at the initial hearing;[422] where a registrant's fitness to practise was impaired by insufficient knowledge of English, lack of competence or health, the panel may not impose strike-off unless the registrant has been continuously suspended or subject to conditions for two years (excluding interim orders).[423]

---

[422] Article 30(1)(b)

[423] Article 29(6)

101.2 Where strike-off becomes available, review hearings assume heightened significance. Practitioners should identify warning signs, commonly including repeated non-attendance, disengagement, or failure to produce evidence over successive reviews. Submissions should address the panel's likely concerns directly and realistically. Escalation is typically driven by disengagement,[424] entrenched lack of insight,[425] persistent non-compliance,[426] or the conclusion that continued restriction serves no purpose.[427]

101.3 Where extension is likely, practitioners should invite the panel to define the purpose of the extension and what is expected before the next review. Decisions will often provide guidance on the progress the panel expects to be made, and how such progress might be measured. Any extension must be justified by reference to ongoing impairment and risk; it is not a neutral outcome.

101.4 Where revocation is sought, submissions should address both safety and proportionality. Panels must justify continued interference with professional life.

[424] See: *Ogbonna-Jacob v Nursing and Midwifery Council* [2013] EWHC 1595 (Admin), at [14]

[425] See: *Unozor v Nursing and Midwifery Council* [2016] 2 WLUK 667

[426] See: *Arora v General Medical Council* [2012] EWHC 1560 (Admin), at [25]

[427] See: *Abbas v Nursing and Midwifery Council* [2019] EWHC 971 (Admin)

CHAPTER ELEVEN

RESTORATION HEARINGS

102 **Purpose**

102.1 Restoration is the statutory mechanism by which a registrant who has been struck off may, in principle, return to practice. It is not an appeal against the striking-off decision and not an opportunity to re-litigate the original findings. The question for the panel is whether, at the date of the restoration hearing, the applicant has demonstrated that they now meet the requirements for admission and are a fit and proper person to practise, having particular regard to the circumstances which led to removal.

103 **Statutory framework**

103.1 The restoration jurisdiction is governed by Article 33,[428] with FTP rule 25 applying to the format of the hearing.

103.2 An application may not be made until five years after the striking-off order took effect,[429] and only one application may be considered in any twelve-month period.[430] A striking-off order may also be reviewed where new evidence becomes available after the order is imposed. In such circumstances, the

[428] *The Nursing and Midwifery Order 2001*

[429] Article 33(2)(a)

[430] Article 33(2)(b)

review is to be treated as an application for restoration.[431] Except in the case of new evidence applications, the Registrar must refer an application for restoration to the FTP committee which imposed the order.[432] That is, the committee as a body; not a requirement that the same panel consider restoration as imposed strike-off.[433] In all cases, the applicant must be given an opportunity to appear and argue their case.[434]

103.3 The panel of the FTP committee must not grant restoration unless it is satisfied that the applicant meets the usual requirements for admission to the register and, having regard in particular to the circumstances of the striking-off, is a fit and proper person to practise.[435]

104 Scope of a restoration hearing

104.1 A restoration hearing is forward-looking. The findings of fact and determinations that led to striking-off are final and binding unless set aside on appeal. The panel has no jurisdiction to revisit their correctness and is concerned "*solely* with the question of whether [the applicant] should be reinstated to the Register, having regard to the requirements set out in Art 33 of the 2001 Order."[436] "The central question thus for the committee and the purpose of their deliberations under this regime [has] to be the question whether the practitioner [is] safe

---

431 Article 30(7)

432 Article 33(3)

433 *Balamoody v Nursing and Midwifery Council* [2009] EWHC 3235 (Admin), at [11]

434 Article 33(4)

435 Article 33(5)

436 *Jerry v Nursing and Midwifery Council* [2025] EWHC 2814 (Admin), at [31] (original emphasis)

to practise."[437] Attempts to re-argue the original case, whether directly or indirectly, are therefore misconceived and shall be treated as evidence of limited insight.

105 **Procedure**

105.1 Restoration hearings follow the structure prescribed by FTP rule 25. The presenter opens by setting out the background and directing the panel to relevant determinations.[438] The applicant then adduces evidence relied upon.[439] The panel deliberates and disposes of the application under Article 33, giving reasons.

105.2 The burden lies on the applicant. Fitness to practise is not presumed to revive with the passage of time. The applicant must satisfy the committee, on the balance of probabilities, that they have changed. In practice this requires cogent, consistent and corroborated evidence.

105.3 The applicant will almost always give oral evidence. Insight is central. Panels are entitled to expect applicants to recognise the seriousness of the misconduct that led to striking-off, to understand its impact, and to demonstrate a sustained change in attitude and behaviour. Panels test insight through questioning and are alert to minimisation, deflection and attempts to reopen factual disputes.

105.4 Remediation must be targeted and cogently evidenced. Generic training and reflection are rarely accorded weight unless they address the underlying causes of the misconduct. Panels are

---

[437] *Balamoody,* at [13]

[438] FTP rule 25(2)(a)

[439] FTP rule 25(2)(b)

concerned with what the applicant has actively done to change, not simply with the passage of time.

105.5 Independent evidence is often useful. Detailed testimonials from employers or supervisors who understand the regulatory history, evidence of trust and responsibility in post-removal roles, and coherent employment histories carry significant weight. The absence of such evidence is frequently fatal.

106 Outcomes

106.1 The available outcomes are restoration or refusal. In making a restoration order, the panel may impose requirements as to education, training or experience,[440] and may make a conditions of practice order on restoration.[441]

106.2 A refusal, or the imposition of requirements, is appealable to the High Court.

106.3 Where a second or subsequent restoration application is made unsuccessfully, a panel may direct an indefinite suspension of the right to re-apply.[442] An applicant may seek a review of that direction after three years have elapsed.[443]

---

[440] Article 33(6)

[441] Article 33(7)

[442] Article 33(9)

[443] Article 33(10)

MORE BOOKS BY
LAW BRIEF PUBLISHING

A selection of our other titles available now:-

'A Practical Guide to Probation Breaches and Other Applications' by Mark Thomas
'A Practical Guide to Remarriage and Divorce' by Cordelia Williams & Claire Howard
'A Practical Guide to Privacy, Transparency, Reporting Restrictions and Closed Proceedings in the Court of Protection' by Laura Mannering
'Beaumont on Barristers – A Guide to Defending Disciplinary Proceedings (Second Edition)' by Marc Beaumont
'A Practical Guide to Payments for Environmental Services' by Ben Sharples
'A Practical Guide to the Law of Pregnancy and Maternity at Work' by Rebecca Thomas
'A Practical Guide to Redundancy – Second Edition' by Philip Hyland & Collette Moore
'A Practical Guide to International Issues for Scottish Family Lawyers' by Susie Mountain, Donna McKay, Ken MacDonald
'A Practical Guide to the Law on Deprivation of Liberty' by Ben Troke
'A Practical Guide to Rights over Airspace and Subsoil – Second Edition' by Daniel Gatty
'A Practical Guide to the Law in Relation to Inquests' by Ramya Nagesh
'A Practical Guide to the Construction and Rectification of Wills and Trust Instruments (Second Edition)' by Edward Hewitt
'A Practical Guide to Data Protection in Social Housing' by Clare Paterson
'A Practical Guide to Spousal Maintenance – Second Edition' by Liz Cowell
'A Practical Guide to International Parental Child Abduction Law (England and Wales)' by Dr Onyója Momoh
'A Practical Guide to Deprivation of British Citizenship' by Sean Ell
'A Practical Guide to Commercial Property Service Charges' by Rachel Garton
'A Practical Guide to Clinical Negligence – Third Edition' by Geoffrey Simpson-Scott (Geoff)
'A Practical Guide to the Rights of Grandparents in Children Proceedings – Second Edition' by Stuart Barlow

'The Electronic Communications Code: A Practical Guide – Second Edition' by Kerry Bretherton KC, James Castle, Mark Loveday
'A Practical Guide to the Independent School Standards – September 2023 Edition' by Sarah McKimm
'A Practical Guide to Estate Administration and Crypto Assets' by Richard Marshall
'A Practical Guide to Parental Alienation in Private and Public Law Children Cases' by Sam King QC & Frankie Shama
'Contested Heritage – Removing Art from Land and Historic Buildings' by Richard Harwood QC, Catherine Dobson, David Sawtell
'The Limits of Separate Legal Personality: When Those Running a Company Can Be Held Personally Liable for Losses Caused to Third Parties Outside of the Company' by Dr Mike Wilkinson
'A Practical Guide to Transgender Law' by Robin Moira White & Nicola Newbegin
'A Practical Guide to 'Stranded Spouses' in Family Law' by Mani Singh Basi
'A Practical Guide to Residential Freehold Conveyancing' by Lorraine Richardson
'A Practical Guide to Pensions on Divorce for Lawyers' by Bryan Scant
'A Practical Guide to Challenging Sham Marriage Allegations in Immigration Law' by Priya Solanki
'A Practical Guide to Digital Communications Evidence in Criminal Law' by Sam Willis
'A Practical Guide to Legal Rights in Scotland' by Sarah-Jane Macdonald
'A Practical Guide to New Build Conveyancing' by Paul Sams & Rebecca East
'A Practical Guide to Inherited Wealth on Divorce' by Hayley Trim
'A Practical Guide to Practice Direction 12J and Domestic Abuse in Private Law Children Proceedings' by Rebecca Cross & Malvika Jaganmohan
'A Practical Guide to Confiscation and Restraint' by Narita Bahra QC, John Carl Townsend, David Winch
'A Practical Guide to the Law of Forests in Scotland' by Philip Buchan
'A Practical Guide to Health and Medical Cases in Immigration Law' by Rebecca Chapman & Miranda Butler
'A Practical Guide to Bad Character Evidence for Criminal Practitioners by Aparna Rao
'A Practical Guide to Extradition Law post-Brexit' by Myles Grandison et al
'A Practical Guide to Hoarding and Mental Health for Housing Lawyers' by Rachel Coyle

'Stephens on Contractual Indemnities' by Richard Stephens
'A Practical Guide to the EU Succession Regulation' by Richard Frimston
'A Practical Guide to Solicitor and Client Costs – Second Edition' by Robin Dunne
'Constructive Dismissal – Practice Pointers and Principles' by Benjimin Burgher
'A Practical Guide to Religion and Belief Discrimination Claims in the Workplace' by Kashif Ali
'A Practical Guide to the Law of Medical Treatment Decisions' by Ben Troke
'Fundamental Dishonesty and QOCS in Personal Injury Proceedings: Law and Practice' by Jake Rowley
'A Practical Guide to the Law in Relation to School Exclusions' by Charlotte Hadfield & Alice de Coverley
'A Practical Guide to Divorce for the Silver Separators' by Karin Walker
'The Right to be Forgotten – The Law and Practical Issues' by Melissa Stock
'A Practical Guide to Planning Law and Rights of Way in National Parks, the Broads and AONBs' by James Maurici QC, James Neill et al
'A Practical Guide to Election Law' by Tom Tabori
'A Practical Guide to the Law in Relation to Surrogacy' by Andrew Powell
'A Practical Guide to Claims Arising from Fatal Accidents – Second Edition' by James Patience
'A Practical Guide to Asbestos Claims' by Jonathan Owen & Gareth McAloon
'A Practical Guide to Stamp Duty Land Tax in England and Northern Ireland' by Suzanne O'Hara
'A Practical Guide to the Law of Farming Partnerships' by Philip Whitcomb
'A Practical Guide to the Law of Unlawful Eviction and Harassment – Second Edition' by Stephanie Lovegrove
'A Practical Guide to Costs in Personal Injury Claims – Second Edition' by Matthew Hoe
'A Practical Guide to the General Data Protection Regulation (GDPR) – Second Edition' by Keith Markham
'A Practical Guide to Working with Litigants in Person and McKenzie Friends in Family Cases' by Stuart Barlow
'Protecting Unregistered Brands: A Practical Guide to the Law of Passing Off' by Lorna Brazell
'A Practical Guide to Secondary Liability and Joint Enterprise Post-Jogee' by Joanne Cecil & James Mehigan

'A Practical Guide to the Pre-Action RTA Claims Protocol for Personal Injury Lawyers' by Antonia Ford
'A Practical Guide to Neighbour Disputes and the Law' by Alexander Walsh
'A Practical Guide to Coercive Control for Legal Practitioners and Victims' by Rachel Horman
'A Practical Guide to the Law of Driverless Cars – Second Edition'
by Alex Glassbrook, Emma Northey & Scarlett Milligan
'A Practical Guide to TOLATA Claims' by Greg Williams
'A Practical Guide to Elderly Law – Second Edition' by Justin Patten
'A Practical Guide to Responding to Housing Disrepair and Unfitness Claims' by Iain Wightwick
'A Practical Guide to the Law of Bullying and Harassment in the Workplace' by Philip Hyland
'How to Be a Freelance Solicitor: A Practical Guide to the SRA-Regulated Freelance Solicitor Model' by Paul Bennett
'A Practical Guide to Prison Injury Claims' by Malcolm Johnson
'A Practical Guide to Advising Clients at the Police Station' by Colin Stephen McKeown-Beaumont
'A Practical Guide to Antisocial Behaviour Injunctions – Second Edition' by Iain Wightwick
'Practical Mediation: A Guide for Mediators, Advocates, Advisers, Lawyers, and Students in Civil, Commercial, Business, Property, Workplace, and Employment Cases' by Jonathan Dingle with John Sephton
'The Mini-Pupillage Workbook' by David Boyle
'A Practical Guide to Crofting Law' by Brian Inkster
'A Practical Guide to the Law of Domain Names and Cybersquatting' by Andrew Clemson
'A Practical Guide to the Law of Gender Pay Gap Reporting' by Harini Iyengar
'NHS Whistleblowing and the Law' by Joseph England
'Employment Law and the Gig Economy' by Nigel Mackay & Annie Powell
'A Practical Guide to Noise Induced Hearing Loss (NIHL) Claims' by Andrew Mckie, Ian Skeate, Gareth McAloon
'An Introduction to Beauty Negligence Claims – A Practical Guide for the Personal Injury Practitioner' by Greg Almond
'Intercompany Agreements for Transfer Pricing Compliance' by Paul Sutton
'Zen and the Art of Mediation' by Martin Plowman
'A Practical Guide to Adoption for Family Lawyers' by Graham Pegg

'A Practical Guide to Industrial Disease Claims' by Andrew Mckie & Ian Skeate
'A Practical Guide to Conducting a Sheriff Court Proof' by Andrew Stevenson
'A Practical Guide to Vicarious Liability' by Mariel Irvine
'A Practical Guide to Applications for Landlord's Consent and Variation of Leases' by Mark Shelton
'A Practical Guide to Relief from Sanctions Post-Mitchell and Denton' by Peter Causton
'A Practical Guide to Equity Release for Advisors' by Paul Sams
'A Practical Guide to Financial Services Claims' by Chris Hegarty
'A Practical Guide to Financial Ombudsman Service Claims' by Adam Temple & Robert Scrivenor
'A Practical Guide to Running Housing Disrepair and Cavity Wall Claims – Second Edition' by Andrew Mckie & Ian Skeate
'A Practical Guide to Holiday Sickness Claims – Second Edition' by Andrew Mckie & Ian Skeate
'Arguments and Tactics for Personal Injury and Clinical Negligence Claims' by Dorian Williams
'A Practical Guide to Drone Law' by Rufus Ballaster, Andrew Firman, Eleanor Clot
'On Experts: CPR35 for Lawyers and Experts' by David Boyle
'An Introduction to Personal Injury Law' by David Boyle

These books and more are available to order online direct from the publisher at www.lawbriefpublishing.com, where you can also read free sample chapters. For any queries, call us on 0844 587 2383 or email us at mail@lawbriefpublishing.com.

Our books are all generally in stock at www.amazon.co.uk with free next day delivery for Prime members, and at good legal bookshops such as Wildy & Sons.

We are regularly launching new books in our series of practical day-to-day practitioners' guides. Visit our website and join our free newsletter to be kept informed and to receive special offers, free chapters, etc.

You can also follow us on Twitter at www.twitter.com/lawbriefpub.

www.ingramcontent.com/pod-product-compliance
Lightning Source LLC
LaVergne TN
LVHW052312200926
848481LV00002B/537